THE METABOLIC
MIRACLE

Work edited in collaboration with Editorial Planeta – Colombia

Original title: *El milagro metabólico*

Translated from the Spanish by Azzam Alkadhi

© 2021, Carlos Alberto Jaramillo

© Editorial Planeta Colombiana S. A. – Bogotá, Colombia

Derechos reservados

© 2021, Editorial Planeta Mexicana, S.A. de C.V.
Bajo el sello editorial PLANETA M.R.
Avenida Presidente Masarik núm. 111,
Piso 2, Polanco V Sección, Miguel Hidalgo
C.P. 11560, Ciudad de México
www.planetadelibros.com.mx
www.paidos.com.mx

Cover design: Grupo Planeta Art Department

First edition printed: September 2021
ISBN: 978-607-07-8167-4

This book was printed in Impresora Tauro, S.A. de C.V.
Año de Juárez Av. No. 343, Granjas San Antonio,
Iztapalapa, C.P. 09070, Mexico City
Printed and made in Mexico / *Impreso y hecho en México*

Dr. Carlos Jaramillo

THE METABOLIC MIRACLE

Eat well, control your weight and turn your body into your closest ally

 Planeta

Contents

For Adriana, for Luciano and
my parents, of course

Prologue
By Dr. Santiago Rojas

Metabolism and its functioning are the hot topic in science today, with a need to understand the origin and find possible solutions to the most common health issues among inhabitants of this new millennium. Investigative evidence on this topic reveals that our current lifestyle has serious repercussions for the working of our metabolism. Bad eating habits and a hectic lifestyle, among other things, force our organism to travel along unnatural paths which, sooner or later, result in ailments of all sorts, and even serious illnesses. Hence the increase in rates of obesity, fatigue, stress, anxiety, insomnia, depression, diabetes, cancer, and autoimmune and cardiovascular diseases, among many other illnesses. But not everything is lost: understanding the origin of the problem will give us the key to modifying those effects.

Understanding begins with an assumption that each one of us is responsible for our own wellbeing, avoiding the feeling of being a defenseless victim of a system which creates, fosters and strengthens poor health and, on the contrary, making up an active part of the solution. That is why I find this work by Doctor Carlos Jaramillo essential. At a time when there is an overwhelming excess of information on the topic of metabolism, diets and health, it is necessary to have clear and conclusive answers like those revealed in this book.

In *The metabolic miracle*, the author not only shares a solution which is applicable to everyone's life, but also dismantles the myths and false beliefs (largely fostered by the food industry and the medical discipline itself) which have led us to the current age of general poor health. With this book the readers will understand the process leading to the rise illness or health. Altogether more importantly, you will receive the necessary tools for changing your life habits and starting to enjoy the benefits of this transformation. You will feel encouraged to convert theoretical learning into a daily exercise, in which, day by day, you make the correct choices in favor of your health.

The deep understanding that the reader will get from these pages, and the inspiration they will gain from taking charge of themselves are two of the great achievements of this book. Two innovative aspects which will facilitate the improvement of our individual health and, in consequence, will also help to modify society in a substantial way. That way, we will give life to our years and give many more years to our lives.

Thank you Carlos for your constant search for knowledge and the generous drive which leads you to share what you know with all those who want to learn from it. This work is the result of that effort and I am sure that it will achieve its aim.

Dr. Santiago Rojas
BOGOTA, FEBRUARY 2019

Introduction
The medicine of the future

It was almost 3:00 in the morning on a day in August, 2011. It was my last shift as a resident in general surgery. I had studied Medicine because I wanted to be a surgeon; I wasn't interested in any other specialty. That had always been my dream. But that morning, as I drank a horrible, sugary coffee at the nurse's station on the sixth floor of a well-known Bogotá hospital, I gazed despondently at the letter tending my resignation from that institution, where I had spent the last two years of my life. My glittering dream had become a painful story.

That early morning, I was filled with dread. I was saying goodbye. I would no longer be a surgeon. What the heck was I going to do? How could I be of use? My internal fears manifested themselves every day, every week and every month that I continued without direction. The decision I had taken was not popular with my family. At that moment, I went from being the model son to a kind of relative it was best to hide in the attic. With the passing of the years I came to understand that their unease and fear were simply a reflection or projection of my own.

I began a search which took me on a beautiful journey of my internal processes, which helped me understand why I had wanted to be a surgeon. I realized that, as well as operating, I was drawn to: 1) being able to heal people and 2) the delightful world of nutrition, which I had learned about in my days at Yale University, with my teacher and inspiration, the renowned Doctor Stanley Dudrick, creator of parenteral (intravenous) nutrition and perennial Nobel Prize in Medicine candidate. So I looked for a path which would allow me to set these two motivations into practice, and I found it in Functional Medicine. You'll be wondering: " Functional Medi... What?". I'll explain in plenty of detail in the coming pages.

My parents also asked me what it meant when I told them I was going to the United States to study Functional Medicine. "What is that? Have you gone mad? We hope that you don't come back to Colombia barefoot, bearded, wearing a turban and smelling of incense!". You're just getting to know me, so perhaps you want to know the answer. No. No turbans. No incense. **Functional Medicine is a branch of Medicine which looks into the origin of illnesses and not their symptoms.** It wants to find the "root of the problem". If you have a migraine, for example, we have to understand where it came from and how it came about; a functional doctor's solution is not to prescribe some medications and bid you a good afternoon so that the next patient can come on in. Functional Medicine is the medicine of 'why?'. Many of the people I assist explain it in a simpler way: "You 'functionals' hit the nail on the head". That's what we do. Or at least we try. We aren't infallible. Nobody is.

Upon studying Functional Medicine, I understood that diseases don't exist, but dysfunctions do. I understood that human beings are unique in their physiological individuality, their immune biochemistry, their social genetics, among other characteristics. Each patient is a one-off road map. I know the qualities of this discipline because I, myself, was my first patient. After taking omeprazole for 14 years, in an attempt to calm a reflux that had followed me around since childhood, I was able to cure it without pills or potions. I simply put into practice what I had studied. Goodbye omeprazole! So long reflux. That small victory spurred me on to keep learning, investigating, reading and understanding the human body. Since then, I have made those same tools available to the thousands of patients I have seen to and for whom we have found their cure.

There are very few of us South American professionals who have studied Functional Medicine formally in the United States; there are very few of us practicing in the Spanish-speaking world, and there are even fewer who have begun to write about the topic in Spanish. That's why this book is a rarity. I started writing it almost a year ago. And, if I'm not wrong, it is the first to address the issue of curing the metabolism from that perspective and in Spanish.

What is this text about? **In it I'm going to suggest that you set out on your own metabolic healing using the best medication that I know: food. If you know how to choose them, combine it, and understand when you should (or should not) include certain foods in your diet, you will have taken a massive step towards your recovery. It all begins with that choice.** That is the beginning and the end because, as I will explain in the first part of this text, we live in a world made sick by its insatiable appetite, a world that doesn't stop eating, eating badly, eating junk food, eating at all hours of the day, eating with the backing of the sector's large industries who encourage an unhealthy consumption and who want the entire planet to devour their mass-produced packaged and tinned goods, and soft drinks. This way of feeding ourselves has provoked an unstoppable increase in metabolic syndrome illnesses and fatal victims. A sick world, for its part, also benefits another enormous industry, pharmaceuticals, which, for years, supplied me with the omeprazole which I no longer need.

In order for you to be able to alleviate metabolic disorders which cause obesity, high blood sugar levels, elevated cholesterol and triglycerides, among other disorders which, sadly, can lead to a cardiovascular episode, first you need to understand your body better. Here I'll introduce you, in simple terms, to many of the stars of the movie that is your metabolism (hormones, organs, glands), like insulin, leptin, cortisol, uric acid, the liver, the pancreas, the intestine, the stomach, your blood, your brain and body fat, among others; it's a very eclectic cast. If all of these "actors" work harmoniously together, your life will be better. The way you feed yourself will give harmony to each of them.

That's why we are going to thoroughly check the characteristics and traits of the food you eat on a daily basis, the all-too-famous macronutrients: carbohydrates, proteins and fats; healthy ones! And together we are going to dispel a lot of myths and legends which we turn into truths by pure repetition, such as, for example, that breakfast is the most important meal of the day, that if we work out on an empty stomach we will "eat" the muscle, that we should eat every three hours, that all fats clog the arteries, that it is necessary to drink milk so that our bones don't break, that we have to count the calories on every plate... And here's where I begin to get mad because, as I will explain in detail later, calorie counting is of no use at all. And finally, once you've understood the benefits of foodstuffs and how they affect your organism positively or negatively, we will then go over the three most important steps for attaining the metabolic miracle: what to eat (and what not to eat), how to mix those foods, and when to eat them (or simply when not to eat).

That's it in a nutshell. And this is how I write it all, just like these lines you're reading, in a relaxed, simple manner, in the same way that I tend to talk at lectures, in sessions with my patients, chatting with my friends, and in much the same way that I frequently give advice on my social media pages, especially my Instagram account (@drcarlosjaramillo).

Today, when I look back on that morning when I was drinking that bad coffee and giving up my *Grey's Anatomy* surgeon's life, I give thanks to life for opening up another path for me. Today I really am living my dream. Today I practice the type of medicine I always wanted to and which allows me to correct chronic illnesses in those who walk into my practice, illnesses that, in the lecture halls of traditional medicine, they told me could not be cured (like diabetes). Today I give my patients the best medicine of all, I teach them that they don't need medicine, I explain to them that, in each and every one of us lives the power of healing. Today, from the love of my son Luciano, I work for the health of children, child nutrition and to educate mothers and fathers so that they can be the pillar of healing in their home. I practice the medicine of the future, but in the present.

NOTE

The information provided in this book is of informational purposes only, and should not be used as a substitute for medical prescriptions, diagnoses or treatment. Neither the author or the publishing house assume responsibility for damages caused by the omission of this warning.

Part one

The metabolic problem

Chapter 1

The epidemic

The global health model has to change. As Chris Kresser explains in his book, *Unconventional Medicine* (2017), it is believed that our children could make up the first generation to live shorter lives than their parents. I agree with his assertion and it worries me. The main cause of this disaster, and of millions of deaths around the world, is metabolic disease. I don't mean to sound like a pessimist, but every day in my clinic I see patients of all ages with metabolic syndrome. The evidence is there, but it would appear that we don't want to see it, or that some large and powerful multinational companies don't want us to see it. This is a problem which involves you, your family, your friends, the people that you care about and people you know. It concerns us all.

But let's start at the beginning: what is metabolism? According to what our dear Aunt Bertha —I'm picking a name at random— once told us, it's a trait which allows human beings to go to the toilet every day to get rid of whatever our organism doesn't need.

What's more, as she would explain, there are two types of metabolism: fast and slow. The former is the "good" one, a blessing reserved for skinny people. The latter is the "slow" one, a divine (and genetic) curse which makes people obese. Yet Aunt Bertha, as sweet as she is, was wrong. That's why I'm asking you to forget these notions, which, by the way, are firmly rooted in the collective imagination.

I put to you a simpler definition: metabolism is the capability of the body's cells to properly use the oxygen and nourishment which enter the organism in order to produce energy. A part (or organelle) of our cells, called the mitochondrion, is vital to this process. This will sound familiar to you, because we were all told about them in biology class at school. There are millions of mitochondria in the human body. Some organs, like the heart and the brain, carry 70 % of them, because they need to constantly produce energy. If oxygen and food are our sources of energy, if they are vital to our metabolic process, then you'll understand the importance of every little piece of food that makes its way into your mouth, right?

However, over the last fifty years, our eating habits have undergone a dramatic, non-beneficial transformation, causing the increase in number of patients with metabolic syndrome across the world. Obesity is growing at an alarming rate, just take a look at the news. If we compare current figures with those from the eighties, we'll see that cases of diabetes have quintupled, as indicated by World Health Organization (WHO) reports. Today it is estimated that one in five, or even two in three, adults on earth —depending on the country they live in— could have diabetes or prediabetes, and this is a huge problem.

But when did this shift begin and how did it come about? In 1950, thanks to advancements and improvements in medical technology, a number of anatomy studies were carried out, which revealed that, in the clogged arteries of various patients, there were deposits of fat. Fat! A word which, from that moment, would become the protagonist in the nightmares of most of humanity. This fear was heightened by an investigation titled the *Seven Countries Study*, published in 1958 by the American biologist and physiology doctorate holder, Ancel Keys. The document, which became a sort of food bible around the world, was the result of many years' worth of research which, unfortunately, left many failed conclusions. Many critics of Keys' work have pondered why, if studies were carried out in over twenty countries, only seven were included in his final text, which took into account demographic groups in the United States, the Netherlands, Greece, Italy, Finland, the former Yugoslavia and Japan.

In his essay, the investigator showed that, in the countries where the greatest quantities of fat were consumed, there were also a higher number of cardiovascular diseases. And on the opposite, in those countries where fat consumption was low, there were fewer such conditions. His conclusions were supported by the anatomical and histological studies of the time, which involved dissecting obstructed arteries, looking at them in the dissection hall and examining them under a microscope. Many of these investigations revealed that there were fatty deposits in these arteries. As a result, for this American biologist, the main global dietary problem was exactly that: the excess of fat.

Was Keys right? No, and we will talk in depth about that throughout the pages of this book, but his investigation had an enormous and, unfortunately, disastrous reach. His theories resounded in a number of media outlets of the time. The investigator appeared on the cover of *Time* magazine on January 13, 1961, in an issue dedicated to "diet and health". The issue shared the dietary blueprint that he was proposing, which was made up of 2,300 daily calories and was based, mainly, on carbohydrates like sugar, pasta, potatoes, bread and fruit, which contributed to 69 % of this diet. This is how it was laid out on page 49 of the magazine. Today, his proposal sounds absurd, but at the time many people believed it and, worse still, a large part of the Western world's dietary model was based on it. It's very possible that, in some mysterious way, that diet did work for Keys, who passed away in November 2004, two months before turning one hundred.

Doubt will always remain as to why his investigation only included the dietary habits of the populations of seven countries. Why were the other nations studied excluded from his text? Was there some kind of pressure from the pharmaceutical or food industry to do so? Keys took the answers with him to the grave. The only thing we know for sure is that, since the *Seven Countries Study*, the way we eat changed forever.

The celebrity biologist's findings acted as a basis for other studies carried out in 1967, 1969 and 1970, which resulted in the publication, in 1977, of the *Dietary Goals for the United States* document, also known as the "McGovern Report". The text begins with a piece of advice: "These recommendations, based on the most recent scientific evidence, should serve as a guide for each of you to make decisions about your own diet". The intention was probably not bad, but the advice given reinforced the idea that fats are humankind's worst enemy and nightmare, while carbohydrates are the species' savior. But no!

From that moment, the food industry's craze for removing fat from food products began, but when this essential component is removed, food tastes terrible, it tastes like cardboard. So the world's large food companies asked themselves: "what can we do to improve the taste of our products? If they taste bad nobody is going to buy them". And then some genius came up with the solution: "Let's just add sugar!". In that instant, the lives of millions of people across the planet began to change, and the great sugar empire —behind which there are many economic interests, you just need to look at the power it holds in countries like Colombia —began, as well as the persecution of those diabolical fats.

Once the matter of taste was resolved, there was still another issue to deal with: calories. If you do a quick check on the world of macronutrients, made up of proteins, carbohydrates and fats, you will find that the first two contribute four kilocalories per gram, while the latter contributes a little over double, nine kilocalories per gram, such that, apparently, if the "evil" fats contain so many calories, then the dietary problem on a global level must be directly related to them. And that's how this brilliant conclusion was reached: 1) If fats clog arteries, 2) and fats contain more calories, then 3) the number of calories in our diets must be reduced! That's when the Third World War, the battle against calories, began. For that we have Keys, and the studies of the time which were based on his conclusions, to thank. Thus the sugar empire began to grow and, with it, diabetes, obesity and many, many other diseases.

The famous British nutritionist John Yudkin (1910-1995) wrote one of the best texts on the subject in 1972: *Pure, white and deadly: how sugar is killing us and what we can do to stop it*. What a title! Amazing, right? This is a book which is rarely cited, and which it appears the large food companies prefer to keep hidden, due to its revealing conclusions. I recommend you read it, you can pick it up at your favorite online store or find extracts online. Yudkin masterfully describes all of the problems which sugar brings.

Our daily bread

Going back to the start, this has to change. We're doing badly. The planet is doing badly. Medicine boasts many technological advancements, with progress in robotics, in diagnostic imaging, in surgical devices; every day there is a new molecule replacing another one, which itself had replaced the previous one. Do you have gastritis? Take omeprazole. Didn't work? Then try esomeprazole. Do you want something else? There's lansoprazole. Not that? Look, here's the latest: pantoprazole. The system's idea is just that, for you to forget your old medication and switch it for a more advanced one, although at the end of the day it's a variation on what you already know.

The industry insists on investing more and more money in order to keep inventing the same thing. That's the state of our current health system and it leads nowhere. **Yes, we're living longer, but we're living worse. We've extended the life expectancy the world over, but at what cost? The price we are paying is too high. Medical advancements guarantee us a longer existence, but if we examine things, we find that chronic illnesses are affecting us earlier and earlier.** As you read this, the laboratories will already have invented another super-new molecule.

Since the seventies, the fear of fats hasn't stopped growing. This dread expanded thanks to the conclusions of the investigations I mentioned paragraphs ago. From that point, diets which are low in fat and high in carbohydrates were introduced. The theory indicated that the latter should be our main source of energy. In other words, glucose was the essence of life. Pure fuel. The body's petrol. Yes, Daddy Yankee, that was the motto of the time: *"Dame más gasolina"* (Give me more gasoline). More sugar!

To reinforce this idea, in 1992 the United States Department of Agriculture (USDA) presented its famous food pyramid. And if we were already going badly, with these new suggestions everything went to pot. The recommendation was clear, and wrong: it stated that a person should eat between six and eleven portions of carbohydrates a day. Here's an image of the damned food pyramid from the early nineties so that you can study it carefully.

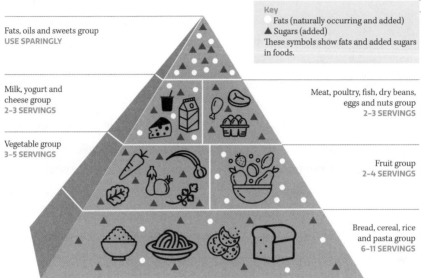

I think the image is pretty clear. Just look at the base of the pyramid. According to this recommendation, we would all need to include in our diet between six and eleven portions of pasta, potatoes, cassava (yucca), biscuits and cereals, including breakfast cereals. In other words, sugar and gluten. Then, we find fruits and vegetables; next up, meat, dairy products, eggs and nuts. And finally, sweets, oils and the condemned fats. At the time it was claimed that this was the way to make our diet more balanced —although it was a lie. Behind all of these ideas were the United States' large food companies—. All of them happily participating and telling people: "That's right, consume our products!".

It's worth noting that, at the time, there had been a huge growth in the corn industry. Breakfast cereals began to make their presence in the breakfasts of millions of families across the world. It was a very easy routine: buy a box of *flakes*, take it to the table, serve it, eat quickly and you're done. Some brands even won over children with figurines or drawings from their favorite comic strips. And a lot of people also ate these cereals for lunch and dinner.

Another beneficiary was the baked goods sector because, of course, the first rung of the pyramid clearly suggested that we needed bread. A lot of bread. Therein was a large part of the "energy of life". Bread and cereals, that's what we were supposed to be giving our kids. We all ate them, and we all liked them; me included. But did following this diet do us any good? In any case, the large multinationals didn't really care, they managed it by creating new products with more colorants and more sugar so that we would all be "happy".

But we were still missing the icing on the cake. In 1995, the American Heart Association (AHA), published a pamphlet with its dietary recommendations, and declared that we should all eat six or more servings of cereals, bread, starchy vegetables (potato, yucca, plantain, sweet potato, among others) because these were low in fat and cholesterol. Not content with this advice, they suggested we drink fruit juices and punches, even soft drinks. It sounds unbelievable, I know, but it's true. The world's most respected cardiology institution, and the one which all of the branch's specialists use as a guide, making such suggestions turned out to be disastrous. Bread and soft drinks. Wow, what geniuses!

The sweet pandemic

Over the last few decades, the numbers for every chronic illness on the planet have increased. Every day there is more cancer, more diabetes, more heart attacks. Every day the number of noncommunicable diseases increases, much more than infectious diseases. Before, people lived less, they died younger, but not because of chronic illnesses. Cancer or infections killed them. It wasn't possible to operate. Dying was simple. Perhaps you were down by the river enjoying a sunny day with your family and, unfortunately, you broke a leg, had an open fracture, there were no antibiotics, no way of curing it and you died. And perhaps you hadn't even turned thirty. But those were different times.

Before the invention of antibiotics, the main cause of death around the world was communicable disease, that is to say, infectious diseases. Today, with all of medicine's advancements, the panorama is different, but not altogether more encouraging. Noncommunicable diseases (NCDs) outnumber infectious diseases. On the first of June, 2018, the World Health Organization reiterated that NCDs "kill 41 million people each year, equivalent to 71 % of all deaths globally". Among said diseases, those which take the most victims are cardiovascular diseases, cancer, respiratory illnesses and diabetes.

We live longer, but we don't live better. And every day our children run the risk of making up part of those fatal figures. We can help them, we can avoid it if we take care of their diets. The figures don't lie: each year in the United States, 3,000 cases of strokes in children under the age of ten are reported. **These are children who drink formula, which is riddled with sugar, from birth; who don't stop drinking soft drinks because they are "the spark of life", and who start their day with sugary breakfast cereals. We are creating an army of sugar addict children who will grow up to be sick adults.** But this trend can be changed. And we can all be part of this change. That is one of the main reasons why I am writing the book which you now hold in your hands.

Going back to recent history and the global panorama, I want to talk to you about the case of China. In 1980, just 1 % of the population suffered from type 2 diabetes, also known as "adult-onset diabetes". Today, 11.6 % of the nearly 1.4 billion inhabitants of the Asian giant have this disease (more or less 160 million citizens). Since 2007, more than 22 million diabetics have added to this figure in the country, a number very close to the entire population of Australia! In just one generation, the numbers for this disease in the People's Republic of China increased by 1,160 %. You read that correctly. It sends shivers down my spine. What was the reason behind diabetes increasing at such an alarming rate? The dietary changes in the country, thanks to the mass arrival in the country of the Western poison: sugar.

It's not just China. On a global level, the problem isn't getting better. Studies indicate that, between 2020 and 2030, one in three Americans will have diabetes. And by 2040, one in every 10 people on the planet will suffer from it.

It's a "sweet" pandemic which has no respect for culture, gender, religion, race or class.

That's how it is. Diabetes, cardiovascular diseases, strokes and heart attacks are increasing around the world. And all those maladies are directly related to our diet, even if we don't want to see it or understand it. We prefer to believe what tradition dictates or what our family physician tell us: that it's a "genetic problem". High cholesterol? Surely someone in your family had it and you inherited it. No family member had it? Ah, then your mother-in-law must have infected you via hypnosis. **We have to set aside the belief that all health problems are hereditary and that our genetic information is like a curse that repeats itself generation after generation. The real enemy is our lifestyle. It's not our genes' fault.**

One of the investigators who helped to decode the human genome (at the beginning of this century) was asked if he considered these revelations a success. He answered that, if by success we meant achieving the complete decoding of this DNA chain, then yes. But if "success" is measured by the ability to explain specifically what this discovery was useful for, then no; these findings had achieved little.

I would say that they were useful in making us realize that we are very similar to rats. Almost identical. That's how a study, which came out in *Nature* magazine in 2004, explained it. Ninety percent of the genes of these rodents have a "more or less evident" connection to ours. We live our lives based on a bunch of genes which, of course, do demonstrate genetic predispositions to certain diseases, but what they forget to tell us is that this genetic information can be modified. That is what a branch of science called epigenetics is dedicated to. This tells us that, beyond if we have inherited certain genes or not, it is up to our relationship with our surroundings whether they "switch on" or "turn off" (like Christmas lights). The bad news is not that we have received them in our inheritance; in the last 4.5 billion years, genetics has hardly changed at all; the bad news is that, with our habits and our lifestyle, we can "switch on" a "defective" gene and clear the way for a disease. But everything —I will say it a thousand times in this book, don't hate me for repeating it, but I will— begins with the diet you choose.

Over the last seventy years, our eating habits have transformed. We have witnessed the boom in plastic packaging, chemicals, preservatives, removing fat from products, the introduction of sugars, the widespread increase in artificial colorings and flavorings, and frozen food. Every day we see the production capacity of the food industry increase. It doesn't matter how harmful the new food this creates is, or how many chemicals it contains to fix the flavor and ensure it's appetizing in Tokyo, New York or Bogota, the industry only cares about producing more, quicker, and spreading its tentacles. Those are the laws of the market. Eat badly, quickly and repeat, that is the invitation being made to us by this industrial blueprint. If you and I accept this junk food, it will do its fatal job in our bodies. It's up to us to say Yes or No, thank you.

The floor is wet

In functional medicine, which is the branch I practice and in which I have specialized —the very same which some medical colleagues discredit and wrongly label "pseudoscience"— we don't focus on the "consequences"; we study and investigate each case in detail in order to try to understand the reason behind our patients' illnesses. It is medicine which asks questions and doesn't cure everything with a pill or predefined prescription, because each person is different.

I like to explain my matter with this example. Imagine that you get home to find the floor in the living room covered in water and you have guests coming in a few hours. The first thing you'll do is deal with the immediate problem, you have to dry the floor. You'll get out several mops and towels, ask for help from your family or even a neighbor, and after a few minutes the floor will be dry. When the guests arrive, it will all just be an anecdote. But the next day, when you get home, the living room floor is flooded again. You repeat the same operation: mop, towels, family, neighbor, done! However, a day later, upon seeing the same problem, you dig a little deeper, find a hole, which is the cause of the leak, and call the plumber and a specialist roofing company, and the problem is solved permanently.

In most cases, traditional medicine follows the first path: it helps the patient dry the living room floor. If it gets wet again, it sends in a couple of drying specialists. If the problem persists, it will send in an army stocked with the latest range of mops to remove every last drop from the floor. And yes, the urgent issue has been resolved. But shortly after, the water will fall to the floor again and the operation will be repeated one, two, a hundred, a thousand times.

Functional medicine takes the second path. There's water in your living room? Ok, let's dry it. But why did it flood? Did you leave a tap running? What could be the cause? Ah, you have a hole in your roof. We need to fix that. This repair might take a few days, but we know what the cause of the problem is and we are working to fix it. Some time later, when you get back home, your living room will be just as you left it, and the roof, better than ever. It's not about more modern mops! It's about finding the source of the leak and making the necessary repair.

It was in the United States that this school of functional medicine was born. Its founding father is Jeffrey Bland (Illinois, 1946), an internal medicine specialist with a doctorate in biochemistry, and my professor at The Institute for Functional Medicine (IFM). He is now somewhat removed from the academy. He started to discover the importance of the intestine and gut flora in the correct functioning of our organism. Bland made a call to attention: he argued that it is the intestine which connects us with the external layer. For example, a skin disease isn't really found on the skin, it is the external manifestation of something internal. A condition affecting the respiratory mucosa is proof that something is happening inside us and does not necessarily have anything to do with the air we are breathing.

He assimilated all of these findings with his knowledge of biochemistry. Thus he found different answers to those being offered by conventional medicine and began to explore other paths. He organized many meetings with some of his friends who were internists, cardiologists, oncologists or colleagues who were working on similar theories. At first his conclusions only provoked laughter, but today he is the creator of a movement which is changing the world and the way in which medicine is practiced.

It didn't happen too long ago. Bland started to develop his investigations at the beginning of the nineties. In 1997 his studies began to be heard and in the first decade of this century, the "great explosion" took place. His revelations have been spread, accepted, studied and continued by renowned professors, doctors and authors, such as Mark Hyman (*Eat fat, get thin*), David Ludwig (*Always hungry!*) and David Perlmutter (*Grain brain*). They are the people I follow, they are my teachers on this path of Functional Medicine, and it's their example which encourages me to continue driving this movement, on the right track and towards a good end. We're not interested in drying the water from the living room floor; we're looking for the holes in the roof and we want to fix them. But it's a complicated task because the planet's medical system is ruled by the law of the mop.

Perhaps you don't know this, but medical associations across the whole world are funded by the food industry or big pharma. And I suppose there must be good intentions from some companies (few), but it's clear that, if they invest in these studies, they don't expect their findings to affect the sales of their products and drugs. The sad thing is that a large part of the "scientific evidence" and "global medical literature" —I used the quote marks deliberately— are being written by "hired specialists", paid for by the multinationals. They will, at the large conferences that bring together those from the profession, and where the latest advancements in medicine are endorsed, give us their half-truths; and they will promote them the planet over. And we keep believing that the correct way to practice our profession is to give more medication to our patients. "Doctor, I've got high cholesterol"; "Take your pill". "Doctor, I have gastritis"; "Here's your little tablet". "Doctor...". There's always a pill to fix anything. A solution that doesn't solve a thing. A top-of-the-range mop for the wet floor. And thus we do little to help those who come to our doctor's offices to heal themselves: we aren't looking for the things that affected their cholesterol or provoked their gastritis; and likewise with other illnesses. We don't see the hole. We don't seal it.

The pharmaceutical companies will be glad because sales of their rescue remedies will increase and their medicines' superpowers will be authenticated by the specialists they support.

Every day millions of people will be buying them, in the same way that they will also invest their money in soft drinks, breakfast cereals, packaged foods and various frozen goods. The food industry has a starring role in this equation of an obese, sick and metabolically-imbalanced world. And of course it will if nobody is capable of stopping it! Whatever happened to the lawsuits filed against a renowned cola drink company for the amount of sugar their drinks contain? Nothing. I remember that the American Beverage Association (ABA) once came out in their defense, claiming that, at the end of the day, human beings need to drink two liters of liquid a day and that we also need some carbohydrates in our diet, which is why sugary drinks exist. The only thing missing was for them to ask us to thank the company for doing such a kind favor for humanity. In their press release on the issue, they said in summation: "We reject any other objection that somebody might have in this regard". Scary stuff.

There have been a lot of similar cases around the world. When they tried to sue a renowned fast food company for promoting bad eating habits, their defense lawyers argued that the brand's icon, a well-known clown, had never invited a child to come and eat hamburgers at its restaurants. The "clown" was just to inspire happiness and joy in children. And there's nothing wrong with that. Or is there?

The other holocaust

Here in Colombia and in many other Latin American countries, it has been very difficult to establish a ruling which allows the consumer to know, in a clear and verified fashion, what is contained in each product they take home. That's why it's worth looking at the example set by nations like Chile. In the southern country, one in every eleven of its citizens' deaths is related to problems of obesity. Faced with these figures, the national government decided to take a more active role in warning buyers about what type of food they would find in their supermarkets. So the Ministry of Health promoted the Food Nutritional Labels Law which it now regulates. This ensures that every packet includes some black circles, emulating a "stop" sign, and on them, in white lettering, reads the warning: "High in". So whoever goes to purchase any food product will know if it is "High in" sugars, sodium, saturated fats or calories. This labelling system was praised in an article in *The New York Times*. It would be worth our while checking it out in this country and across the region.

There's something I find rather odd. When a nation has concrete proof, or even vague indications, that the lives of its inhabitants are at risk —from threat of war, bombing, a wave of immigration—, it is prepared to take the most extreme measures, invading the neighboring country, shooting down suspicious aircraft, taking fire against strangers, killing others to guarantee the lives of our own. But if there's anything that murders more people than the worst armed conflict and has claimed more victims than any genocide, it is the misguided way we feed ourselves, the excess of sugar we consume daily, the terrible health system we have and the lack of awareness of these three things. In most countries, the number of yearly deaths as a result of these things is greater than the number of victims of the Nazi holocaust. But nobody talks about that.

Each year, the budget assigned by the world's nations to their health systems requires more and more investment into treating cases of metabolic syndrome, cardiovascular, cerebrovascular and metabolic diseases. By 2020, it is estimated that one in every three dollars of the United States' health plan will be assigned to treating cardiovascular diseases, diabetes and their complications. The problem is clear: the enemy is right there but we keep attacking it with mops. Do you suffer from diabetes, prediabetes, metabolic syndrome, high cholesterol, obesity? We have some new drugs that will fix it. The medicine didn't work? You had a heart attack or a stroke? No problem, we'll just set up the most cutting-edge intensive care ward for you with all the latest surgical equipment so that we can put in a stent, perform a bypass or perform a bariatric surgery. Afterwards you'll have the best room, the best monitors, a bunch of medication, everything that you need. All the latest technology at your fingertips —if you can afford it, of course—.

Technological advancements have been, and will continue to be, of great help to medicine; their contribution is priceless, but in most cases, what our patients need more than advanced technology is prudent care. I've not seen any health system which makes early interventions when it discovers that citizens have diabetes or high cholesterol. I've not seen one health system which sends those suffering from these problems to consult an appropriate doctor so that, more than simply medicating them, they teach them to identify their problems. I've not seen the first health system which suggests to those patients that they start a tailored training program and look for a good nutritional program, a real one, not those based on calorie counting or reducing fat intake.

Because, and let's be clear about this, a "nutritional program" is not a predefined diet which the on-duty nutritionist keeps in the drawer of their desk and, after adding a stamp and a signature, hands it over to every person they see to. What's needed is a specialist who can recommend a diet based on the needs of each patient. Someone who visits their home —yes, who goes to their house— and identifies those products or habits which might be contributing to their illness. Who looks through their cupboards and fridge and helps them to identify what should stay and what should take a one-way trip to the trash can.

What I'm trying to tell you is that, **before you get to the opera-ting theater equipped with the latest technology, you should make use of the best medicine you have at your disposal: your eating habits. Until this changes, nothing is going to change. Don't forget that** *everything* **that happens in your body is di-rectly related to what you put in your mouth.**

If, for example, you have an injured knee and your daily diet contributes to inflammation in your body, your knee won't get better. If you have an autoimmune disease like lupus, you'll go to the rheumatologist so that they can "cure" you and prescribe you some expensive medication that your insurance will have to approve, and maybe you'll get better that way. But they never tell you that your diet might have been the cause of your illnesses. Nor do they tell you that, if you change your diet under the supervision of a specialist who carefully monitors your progress, your illness, your life, can change. By the way, what did you eat today?

Hippocrates, the father of Medicine, who lived in the fifth cen-tury before Christ, said that whenever a sick person approached him for help, he would always ask them if they were prepared to renounce the causes of their own illness. That is key. However, it's hard for us all to understand that, if we want to cure ourselves of lupus or any chronic complaint, we must modify our lifestyle and change our diet. *All* of the diseases we suffer from —not just cardiometabolic ones— are influenced by our eating habits. Why? Because **food is the information we transmit to our bodies. Each bite and each sip is "data" for our organism. However, we ignore this, or we don't care, because, these days, lunch, breakfast or dinner have become merely the act of eating to fill ourselves up, of eating because we have to, of eating in a hurry because we can't waste time on something so "irrelevant".** It's more im-portant for us to post a tweet on Twitter, a comment on Facebook, or a photo of what we're eating on Instagram than to focus on the actual act of eating. Seen in this way, food becomes a form of cheap energy which enters our body in order to try to get through the hours left each day. And it shouldn't be like this! If food is information, then we need to choose the best information for our organism.

I guarantee that you are more careful with your car's engine than with your own "engine", the one which keeps you alive. If you're told that your new, latest model car only works properly with premium gas, well then you won't fill the tank with diesel fuel, water, cooking oil, sugar or sand. You'll put in the fuel that the mechanic indicated. Otherwise the engine will get damaged. "The car broke down", you'll tell the engineer at the garage. "And are you using the correct fuel?", he'll ask. Well no, that one was really expensive, and I started to use another one mixed with balsamic vinegar", you might respond. "Well, what can I say? It was messed up by idiocy!", the good man will rightly add.

But that's not going to happen. You're very careful with the car; if they tell you to use premium, you'll follow the recommendation down to a T.

Perhaps with your body you don't do the same and you insert any old "mixture". The one that's closest at hand. The one that's cheaper. And that's how the engine fails. It gives your organism the wrong information, it makes it sick; and that's how the epidemic which I'm talking about starts. This will keep spreading unless you wake up and decide to accept the change. In this book I call on you to let us do that together.

How expensive!

Amidst all of this I see positive behavior. Many of my patients and friends speak of their intent to improve their eating habits. People want to eat better —we'll talk in detail about this in the coming chapters—, but they often think that, in order to do so, they will need to invest too much money. Many people say to me: "It's just that those healthy things are really expensive, doctor", but that isn't true. At the end of the day, if we eat badly it's because we choose to do so. The dietary foundation of someone from any social class, regardless of whether they are an omnivore, vegetarian, vegan or if they've chosen to take on the "paleo" diet, should be vegetables, and the majority of these aren't expensive. The distribution of food on our plates, the distribution of nutrients, is basically the same for all human beings, but each of us chooses what to fill the space with.

It's like when you choose your life partner. It doesn't matter what sex, skin color or profession they have, nor if they meet the new millennium's aesthetic prototypes. You fell in love, and so did she (or he). And you've filled a hole with that person you love. You chose.

But you have to make these choices removed from the feeling of separation that's taking hold in the world, apart from the extremes, from the "if you're not with me, you're against me" attitude, because the same thing happens when we talk about people's eating habits. There are culinary Talibans. Meat eaters on a "paleo" diet say that vegans are crazy and a bit stupid; equally, radical vegans, who are now making up a sort of new religion on this planet, furiously take on all those who don't eat like them, and that's the separation I am talking about. It's my way or the highway. But all positions are valid, we all fill the space with what we choose. There is no one path, no one way. I'll try to prove that in the coming chapters.

The solution isn't necessarily to stop eating meat or stop eating something else. No; it's learning to balance what you eat. And that can be done with any economic circumstances, under any dietary regime and in any part of the world. It's also not a question of poverty or wealth; you just need to understand, and set aside the comfort and ease of picking a packet of chips for lunch because you were far from home. Of course, you'll probably wash it down with a soft drink or a juice box and you'll justify it by saying: "I'm hungry and I need to give my body something in order to continue with my day". Or you'll remember old Aunt Bertha's phrase: "If you don't eat, you'll get gastritis". When did they convince you that was true?

Many of my patients arrive at my practice with large envelopes stuffed with medical examinations that various specialists have ordered. Usually the results show that their health is fine. Although the tests suggest that, the majority of patients tend to tell me: "Doctor, I feel really bad". Some are worried about their high cholesterol, others can't lose weight, or have fertility problems or an acne that won't quit, and they've tried everything. However, their test results suggest that they are better than ever. Do the results lie? Are the laboratories failing? No. We as doctors are getting it wrong because we are not looking for the causes, but instead the consequences. And for each consequence, the incredible pharmaceutical industry will have a solution, a pill, a tablet, a powder, the new molecule, which you will take over and over in all of its forms and will forever be a slave to it. What's more, the industry will carry out studies in which it will claim that, by not taking that medicine, you will surely die.

As doctors we fail a lot. We grasp a ton of concepts, we know hundreds of medications, with our diagnostic abilities we can choose the right treatment for our patients, but much of the time we forget to ask ourselves where the illness comes from and what the problem is. Here we are going to try to answer those questions. After reading these pages, you will have the ability to answer them. This book is a tool for you to be able to improve your life. Maybe you'll finally understand that, after mopping the living room thousands of times, what you really need is to patch the hole in the roof. That's the only way.

TEST

HOW'S YOUR METABOLISM?

After having read this first chapter, and understanding that metabolic disorders are very common among the world population and that they can be decisive factors in causing cardiovascular diseases —which are those which cause the most deaths on the planet—, I invite you to answer this questionnaire which will provide us with the first clues on how your metabolism is doing. Shall we begin? You just need to answer, honestly, *yes* or *no*.

	YES	NO
Do you always want to eat?		
If you don't eat at your preset times, do you get angry, get a headache and/or feel dizzy?		
When you're worried, do you get very hungry, or does thinking about food generate anxiety?		
Are you overweight, or do you suffer from adiposity (a little fat, "spare tire", muffin top)?		
Is it hard for you to lose weight in spite of dietary and physical treatments?		
Do you put on weight easily if you don't take care of yourself?		
Do you have a history of hypoglycemia or resistance to insulin?		
Do you or have you suffered from acne?		
Do you have any family history of obesity, overweighting and/or diabetes?		
Do you have high triglyceride levels and/or high cholesterol, low HDL and high VLDL?		
Is the circumference of your abdomen larger than 90 centimeters?		

Do you crave sugar, desserts, pastry and patisserie products, and other wheat products?		
Do you feel bloated and/or do some joints occasionally hurt without apparent reason?		
Have you ever had blood glucose level tests come out higher than 100mg/dL?		
(The following questions only apply to women)		
Do you have a history of ovarian cysts?		
Do you have facial hair or back hair, in the form of fine "lanugo"?		
Are you infertile or have you had a miscarriage?		
Do you have irregular menstrual cycles?		

How many questions did you answer *Yes* to? The higher the number of affirmative responses, the higher the probability of having a metabolic imbalance. However, if your test included lots of yeses, don't be impatient, I suggest you keep reading. This book will serve you by using changes in your diet, your form of exercising, your lifestyle, and by setting aside certain beliefs, to allow you to begin to recover your organism's correct functioning. And you will also set a good example for your family and loved ones.

Chapter 2

The big lie

One of the most common mistakes you can make is thinking of the food that you give your body as simply a summation of calories (I will use the abbreviation CAL to refer to these). Maybe you add them up on your calculator as you sit in front of each dish to see how many you consume every day. I know you've been told you must fight against them, that if there are fewer CAL in each serving, your life will be better. Goodbye obesity and hello health. That's why, following the theory which has become a rule over the past few decades, many people pushed fats aside, because their calorie content is high and, what's more, they are the enemy of man! According to this theory, carbohydrates and proteins will always be the best food source as they contain fewer calories. Based on this reflection, which is false, people started to determine the required calorie count for all human beings on the planet, without thinking that we are all different.

If you're one of those who adds, subtracts, multiplies and divides calories compulsively, I ask you to calmly read this section so that you understand that all of those calculations are not necessary in order to live better.

Let's start at the beginning. What is a calorie? It's simply a unit of energy, period. A food having more or less CAL doesn't make it good or bad. There are CAL which enter your organism get used immediately; others, in contrast, your body leaves in reserve; and there are some which it can't even process or metabolize. When do you burn calories? All the time! What? Yes. In this instant, while you read these lines with your pupils dilated, thinking I'm feeding you a lie, you are burning them; you don't just do it when you go jogging.

Is obesity a result of eating too many calories? It's not that simple. Let's look at it in detail.

We've all been made to believe that fatness is the product of an excess of CAL in our diets. And we're told: "If you eat 500 calories, well then you have to go and burn them". Moms and dads tell their kids that. They warn them that if they want "that dessert", which contains 300 CAL, then later they have to go out and ride their bike —even if it's raining— so that they eliminate those demonic enemies. But our body doesn't work like that, it doesn't operate according to an arithmetic equation of calories that go in and out. Let's say that the math of our body is different. Let's look at it in a simpler fashion with this calculation, and remember it, because we don't work like this:

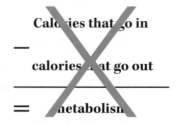

Living beings are NOT the result of this addition and subtraction. That's why calorie counting doesn't work. The mistake is thinking that, if you eat 1,500 CAL, but go to the gym and burn 1,800, you're creating a deficit of 300. You go home happy. You look at yourself in the mirror and say: "I'm winning!". In practice, and this is held up by various studies, this system of adding, subtracting, dividing and multiplying CAL fails in 99.4 % of cases.

Counting calories is a totally dangerous way of thinking because...

1 › It causes people to forget the daily pleasure of eating and only think about how many CAL they are giving to their body.

2 › Worse still, people sit at the table and are madly counting every CAL. Thus, the act of eating and taking in a good meal is replaced by the number being added to a cellphone app which shows how many CAL you have consumed that day. Eating stops being an act of kindness to your body, a time for pleasure and enjoyment. It becomes a moment for a count; a technological count, no less.

3 › Those who count calories with their devices forget another detail: that they are not all the same! We can't say that all carbohydrates are the same, because alcohol, for example, is very different to cookies, broccoli or fruit, which are also carbs. So, dear compulsive calorie counters, it's different eating a hundred CAL of broccoli, candy or cookies, than drinking a hundred CAL of an alcoholic beverage. And the same goes for the other two macronutrients: proteins and fats.

4 › In fact, there are some diets known as *If it Fits Your Macros*, which allow people to fill the space of each one of the macronutrients however they wish. That means that, for example, you can eat chicken (protein), with potatoes and vegetables (carbohydrates), and avocado and olives (healthy fats); or the same chicken, accompanied by jellied candy (bad carbohydrates, full of sugar) and vegetable cooking oil (a non-recommended fat). Notice that they are two different options which could contain the same quantity of macronutrients, but will they give the same information to your body? Of course not! People end up eating junk and only worrying that the number of CAL or servings of "macros" is correct. That is, simply put, absurd.

5 › This obsession with counting calories leads to misled and extreme decisions such as accepting the so-called "cura romana". Those who follow this diet are advised to consume just 500 CAL a day (that is roughly equivalent to eating a chicken breast and two apples in a whole day) and they are injected with a hormone called chorionic gonadotropin. And the specialists will tell them that they have lost weight thanks to the miraculous injection, but how can they not lose weight if they were playing at starvation?

And here I propose another pause. Our organism has a basal metabolic rate. This simply refers to the consumption each of us requires while carrying out normal functions, brain functions, those of the internal organs, breathing, our movements (walking, running, exercise, brushing our teeth). All the time we are burning CAL, even when we sleep. The basal metabolic rate indicates our daily energy outlay. So it therefore sounds logical that, if we do more exercise, we consume more energy and if we also eat less, we will have found the solution to fighting obesity and creating balance in our body. But no! Don't be fooled. It may work initially, but it will not last.

When I talk about this topic I tend to say that, with CAL, the same thing happens as when you receive a pay cut. If you were earning, let's say, 20 dollars, and you were living the good life, going on many trips and eating out at all the city's best restaurants, investing in luxury, top-brand clothing and cutting-edge technology, well it's going to be hard to organize your spending if your salary is suddenly reduced to 10 dollars. Initially it will seem terrible to you; you'll say: "So, no more Armani? No more going out? What a tragedy!". But if you are a prudent person, with the passing of the weeks you will get used to it: you will lower your spending, reorganize your outlays, and you will live with that money. And you can do it with less, no doubt about it. It can always be done. What's more, you could even save a proportion of those 10 dollars after having changed your lifestyle.

Now imagine that I am not talking about your wages, but about your body. It will do the same. If you previously carried out your daily functions using a high number of calories and you start to lower them, your organism will initially start to wonder what's happening —why did they lower my calorie "salary"?—, but with the passing of the weeks you will understand. If you previously used more CAL to breathe, well you can also do it with fewer. The human body is wise and it becomes accustomed. While your body understands it, you, consuming fewer calories, will notice that you lose weight, but when your organism gets used to living "with a lower salary", your weight loss process will end.

And if you want to lose some more pounds and noticed that the strategy worked once before, what will you do? Well, lower your organism's salary even more. Less food! Less CAL! And the process repeats itself. You'll lose weight for a while. But... Exactly! Your body, master of understanding, will once again become accustomed and you will once more say, with a tragic look on your face: "I hit a wall!". However, as you desperately need to drop even more pounds, kilos, or whatever, because you need to get into that dress you like so much in order to go to Laura's wedding, or because you no longer fit in your bullfighter's outfit, you'll start again. Another bodily budget cut. And you'll do it, and keep doing it, and over time you'll understand that is not the solution. If you give your body 500 CAL, it will survive on them.

Now, your body is very intelligent and thrifty. If you consume, for example, 1,500 CAL a day, it won't use up all this calorie content: it will always save a little; it will always have some in reserve and will try to create a balance between the basal metabolic rate —we talked about this a few paragraphs ago— and the resting energy expenditure. It will always be modifying these two variables, increasing or lowering, depending on your metabolism, although sometimes the body can't control the stupid things we do with it.

In my practice, every day I see patients who count their CAL and tell me that they spend two hours working out at the gym and that they literally eat a few lettuce leaves with some water, but they don't lose weight. They bring me all the medical examinations they have been told to undergo. We check them. Everything looks good on the surface, but maybe the tests they were given weren't the ones they really needed, or maybe the clues that lie within those diagnostics have not been properly read. Why? We'll come back to this topic later.

Less is not more

Caloric information is everywhere. On every packet of health food, or of the junkiest of junk food, we will find a notice with the number of CAL it contains. These have been calculated for a standard diet of 2,000 calories. Who decided that was correct? The United States Food and Drug Administration (FDA), based on surveys carried out by the United States Department of Agriculture (USDA). But this is a "model" which doesn't work for everyone in the world. That is to say that, if you are 1.90 meters tall, that number of calories will be low for your needs, but if your height is 1.50 meters, which is the average height of the majority of Latin American women, those 2,000 calories are too many. So everything changes depending on various factors. And not all CAL are the same. Which is why I insist that there are other, more important matters in our diet than damn CAL. I suggest you check some scary evidence: go to the dairy section of the supermarket and pick up one of those yogurts for children or babies. Carefully examine the nutrition facts. How is it possible that the CAL serving in that drink, designed for a six-month old critter, is based on a diet of 2,000 CAL? It's a baby, for God's sake! You can't use the same calculation for everybody.

Numerous investigations have shown that CAL counting does little good. Over many years, at the start of this century, a trial was carried out regarding changes in eating habits in 50,000 women from different ethnic backgrounds in the United States, who took part in the renowned Women's Health Initiative (WHI). This has been, perhaps, the most important and largest study on dietary interventions of its kind. It used detailed parameters to evaluate whether reducing calories worked and if low-fat diets were, in fact, beneficial for the body. In 2006, Doctor Barbara V. Howard presented her findings on what happened with the modification in eating habits of those tested, who subjected themselves to a low-fat diet. What was clear was that the reduction in calories doesn't work and that it's just like appearing in a production of *The Hunger Games*. Furthermore, the WHI's Dietary Modification Trial, which aimed to provide irrefutable proof that fats were the worst thing for the body and that they promoted cardiovascular diseases, in fact did the exact opposite. They found no evidence to support this theory. Following a low-fat diet (less fat, fewer CAL) was of no benefit when trying to avoid this type of disease. We will further develop this idea in another section of the book.

In the long run, a reduction in CAL is going to wreak havoc with the hormones responsible for the proper functioning of our metabolism. That's right, the habit, the obsession with adding and subtracting CAL leads to metabolic disorders. **Daily, I see the suffering of hundreds of my patients starting their marathon against CAL. The worry that not losing weight causes them, despite achieving caloric reduction levels worthy of a hunger strike and having exercise routines akin to Rocky Balboa's, destroys them.** And so the hormones that control their stress levels increase and contribute to them gaining weight, despite their superhuman efforts to lose it. I've seen it. People who consume 500 calories a day and don't manage to get the scales to show the number they want. What's the next step? Anorexia? Bulimia? Stop this adding and subtracting, please.

In 2011 another study was conducted, which investigated the changes in hormones associated with weight loss. Each of the investigation's subjects was given 500 CAL a day which led to a loss of more or less 13.5 kilos. Then they were provided with a diet of low glycemic index carbohydrates, low in fat, and, to maintain these levels, they were asked to exercise for thirty minutes a day. (You can read the study in detail in the analytic article *Long-Term Persistence of Hormonal Adaptations to Weight Loss*, one of the bibliographic references you'll find at the end of this book).

Despite all these interventions, all of the study subjects began to gain weight again. After all that effort, they were putting on the pounds again! The results indicated that several of the hormones being monitored were well above their base levels, especially one of these, ghrelin, the one responsible for sending precise messages to the brain so that we feel hunger.

The study revealed that all of the participants, who were subjected to a diet low in CAL, low in fat, with the best carbohydrates (low in calories), and who followed a strict exercise routine, felt hungrier. Really hungry. And that's a nightmare. A huge number of patients have told me that. Many cry in my practice because they suffer withdrawal symptoms, panic attacks, anxiety crises —because of sugar, in large part—, anxiety about wanting to eat all day. It's not the hunger that is felt in the miserable conditions of poverty which reign in many parts of the world; it's the misery of feeling hunger —despite having it all— because the obsession with counting CAL caused damage to the metabolic system.

This investigation also studied the behavior of other hormones which control fullness, such as neuropeptide Y, amylin and cholecystokinin, which are released in response to the fats and proteins we consume. These hormones help us to feel full. The studies revealed that, after a year, the levels of these hormones were significantly depleted. Summing up, those who took part in this study had high levels of ghrelin, which is why they felt so hungry; and low levels of neuropeptide Y, amylin and cholecystokinin; so it was impossible for them to feel full. It was entirely logical: if they weren't consuming proteins and good fats, they would never feel full. The most discouraging thing was that they were only taking in 500 CAL a day, but they were gaining weight. That is moving towards the worst possible scenario: *The hunger games*, as I said before.

Doctor Ancel Keys, who we spoke about previously, carried out a study in Minnesota called *Starvation*, also known as the Semi-Starvation Experiment. In it, he documented the neurosis caused by hunger in people who lose weight, and who even end up dreaming about food, an effect I have also noticed in those who come into my practice. I understand it more and more. They feel guilty; they say: "Doctor, I don't have enough will power to stop eating". I tell them to free themselves of that guilt, that it's not about "will power"; if they are feeling such intense hunger it is down to their hormonal imbalances. That's what my teacher, Doctor David Ludwig, pediatric endocrinologist at Harvard University, says in his book *Always Hungry* (2016). I've learnt so much from him over the years. That feeling of eternal hunger can overcome the will of even the most disciplined person, of the strongest person.

The guilt that they feel should be shared by us doctors, who do not manage to give the correct solutions to our patients when they need them. We treat them with mops and we don't see their leaks. And we aren't the best example. I say it because I know. When we graduate from med school we have no idea how to nourish ourselves. What a contradiction! We doctors are —supposedly —the ones who know the most about health, but at the same time we are the least healthy people on the planet. We have a terrible lifestyle and awful habits: we don't sleep, we work long shifts, we feed ourselves terribly, we eat to fill ourselves up and get it out of the way, because we are in a hurry, because we need to perform surgery, we need to save lives. However, when our patients arrive, we don't know how to identify anything at all.

Worse still is when dealing with someone who is hospitalized. What diet will they receive in the clinic? Most likely one based on CAL and nutrient counting, regardless of what those may be. Their nature or origin do not matter; if they do not exceed the established values, they will be given to the patient. Maybe it's a liquid diet. Sweet yogurt, jello and fruit juices will be ordered. It's common. However, it's not the most advisable option. Why is someone who has just come out of intensive care, who has spent days battling against large inflammatory processes in their body, given this diet? Why? If sugar inflames the organism! But this is what us medics learn in clinical nutrition classes, though it may seem unbelievable.

Orange–colored stains

Let's resume. In the midst of this CAL reduction competition, pharmaceutical companies saw a new opportunity. If the macron-trients which contribute the most CAL are fats, then they should create a magic pill so that they do not affect people's bodies. That's how Orlistat, which is now prescribed by cardiologists and endo-crinologists from all the medical communities in the world, was born. I'll explain to you what this "beautiful" pill does. If you've enjoyed a fatty feast for lunch, Orlistat will prevent your intestine from absorbing the fat, which will then come out, however fatty it is, in your stool. When you go to the bathroom, you will notice that you have literally expelled an orange-colored oil from your body.

And I don't know if I should talk about the disastrous, terrible and embarrassing effects of this drug. Ok, yes, I will. If you're won-dering how I know them so well, let me tell you: I experienced them first hand, I took Orlistat. Just like many others, I thought it could be a solution. I was wrong. And hopefully my errors will help you avoid repeating the story. I remember it very well, it was in 2006, I was studying medicine and I was given some samples of the medication. I started taking it and the side effects were unfor-gettable. It gave me an uncontrollable urge to go to the bathroom. What's more, as the thousands of people who have taken it will tell you, a gassy expulsion may well be accompanied by some orange droplets which will stain your clothes. It's not pleasant. However, against all logic, Orlistat was named one of the best medications of 2007. A number of studies have been carried out on the drug, some focusing on its efficacy, or lack thereof, at controlling obesi-ty, and its effects on patients with diabetes. Many investigations have revealed that, after four years of taking the pill three times a day, patients ended up putting on the weight that they had lost, and 91 % of them complained about the side effects I mentioned.

I have been able to talk about Orlistat at many forums. At each of these there is always some doctor who comes out with his King Arthur's sword to defend the honor of this medication. They make their declarations about the benefits of the product, defend the caloric reductions to fight obesity and, obviously, shout at the top of their lungs that this pill comes with the Food and Drug Administration's (FDA) approval, as well as that of American medical associations. So I hold my tongue. Everyone will have their orange stains in their underwear moment, a beautiful reminder of science's progress in its fight against fat and calories. I wholeheartedly recommend that you do not buy these pills.

I think you've grasped my message. Throughout these paragraphs I've repeated incessantly the fact that calorie counting *does not* work. As well as the investigations previously mentioned, I know of others which are even more conclusive in their findings. In one of them, the subjects were given a considerable increase in their calorie intake: they reached up to 6,000 per day. Did they gain weight? Here's the most interesting part of the story. Each of the participants received a suitably balanced diet, with an appropriate proportion and type of fats, proteins and carbohydrates. There was a quantitative and qualitative assessment, and a calculation of how much of each food and what kind of food they were given. But I come back to the question: did they gain weight? No. Not one gram. If there's a balance, if we understand how to feed ourselves, if we don't affect the hormones, CAL won't be a problem. That doesn't mean that we can eat excessively; not at all. I am just trying to reiterate that the obsession with calories is not worth it.

We need to stop thinking that our body works like a washbasin, where the water comes out of the tap, falls onto the porcelain and then quickly slips downwards, looking for the plughole, through which it disappears. That's not how calories are eliminated. Don't live for CAL counting, live to enjoy life.

Born to run

On another note, everybody believes that the best way to keep our body in the best state is by exercising. You only need to look as far as one of the most well-received campaigns of Barack Obama's administration, driven by his wife Michelle, the *Let's Move: America's Move to Raise a Healthier Generation of Kids* initiative. The general gist of its proposal was that we should eat less and move more in order to avoid Homer Simpson curves.

The ex-First Lady undoubtedly had very good intentions, but her position reduced the metabolic problem to a mathematical equation: more movement would mean more burnt calories, and therefore we would be healthier. That was the solution: America's kids should move *more*. The initiative spread to schools across the whole country and news clips showed Michelle Obama happily dancing with children and teachers. The kids began to take active breaks; it was a nice effort. Although awareness was raised about the problem of obesity, visibility was given to the topic and it was spoken about around the world, the campaign's results were disheartening. Nothing came of all that dancing. Students continued to gain weight in all of America's schools. But, as it was an Obama plan, and we like them so much, little is said about the failure of their proposal.

A lot of people think the same thing that Michelle Obama did, that the definitive solution to controlling our metabolism can be found in exercise and that those who do not take part will be eternally condemned to have the belly of Bart Simpson's dad. But I just want to remind you that metabolism and an appropriate weight depend approximately 80 % on your diet, and the remaining 20 % on the exercise you do. If you tend to read with a highlighter, I suggest you highlight that. Go on, go and get it, and we'll move on.

I'm not claiming, by any means, that exercising is not important, of course it is, and I am an exercise junkie; I'm just saying that exercising will not give you the magical powers to achieve the metabolic results you're looking for. **Bear in mind that all the exercise in the world could never counteract a bad diet. Highlight that too. You can participate in a thousand marathons, but if your eating habits are poor, it's probable that your metabolism will become unsettled. Many people believe that, because they run five kilometers a day, they can ignore their diet, as if athleticism alone could work miracles. Moving to burn calories, as the Obamas proposed, will not bring an end to the world's metabolic syndrome problems.**

Nor will getting moving, my dear mothers, my dear fathers, make the sugar and CAL that your children are consuming evaporate if you send them to the park to ride their bike. For a child to burn off the calories in a 10 ounce, or 300 milliliter, soft drink, they will need to pedal around on their bike for an hour and fifteen minutes. And if the child also ate a slice of cake at Matthew's birthday party, we'll they'd better devour it while sitting atop their "steel horse", because they are going to have to pedal more than Rigoberto Urán on the Tour de France to dispel that cocktail of calories. That wouldn't be the solution.

Although it's not necessary for us to jump up and down all day and subject ourselves to lengthy gym sessions to achieve metabolic equilibrium, we can't permit ourselves the absurd sedentary routine we live by today either. Let's take a look at our daily activity. We sleep for eight hours —that is to say we are lying down— and then we get up in order to eat our first meal of the day sitting down. Then we travel to work by car, also sitting, in order to arrive at our office where we will spend the majority of our time in that same position. We return home —again, sitting in the car, or on the bus or metro—. When we arrive, we will have dinner —yes, sitting—, and then maybe we will read or watch television lying down, before sleeping our eight hours and following the same routine. That is many people's life cycle. I'm sure that human beings didn't come to the world for that. If that is your case, well then, my friend, it's time to get moving, not to burn calories, but simply to avoid rusting like an old scrap of metal. Exercise and movement are essential to living better. We need to make up for our intellectually-rewarding sedentarism with some daily physical activity. What? Whatever you like, but, please, do it.

Getting back to the main topic of this section, I remember a case which will clearly demonstrate that exercising is not enough to guarantee metabolic equilibrium. It's that of doctor and renowned Canadian surgeon Peter Attia, who is also a great athlete. For many years he exercised intensively and, at some point in his life, despite the hours he had dedicated to training, he had a check-up and realized he had diabetes. Why was he sick if his habits were so healthy? Because Attia was following the diet that became the model in the sporting world. Since the moment we were told that fat was bad and that it clogged our arteries —which isn't true—, we were also assured that the best energy source for our bodies, and especially for those of athletes, came from glucose, which is found in carbohydrates.

It was also claimed that this sped up our body's heat capacity (thermogenesis), raising its temperature and therefore burning more calories. So Attia, like any good athlete, followed a diet which forced him to eat many times a day and which was rich in carbohydrates and glucose! Therefore, despite the large amount of exercise he was doing, he didn't realize that all of the hormones which controlled his metabolism were out of balance. The sad, and worrying, thing is that, even today, that is the dietary model recommended to the majority of athletes in the world. I say it knowingly because I do sports and I also hear these stories from my sporting companions, and it's hard to change their mindset.

Attia is an example of the fact that carbohydrates (and especially the bad ones) are not our organism's savior. They provide energy, but who says that we need to consume them in this way so that our reserves don't deplete? The body doesn't run on a "little tank" which we constantly need to fill up. We aren't old steam trains that need coal or wood all the time; we don't have a gas tank like cars do. Our body's reserves are enormous, but we need to learn to stock them with the right fuel. Peter Attia's mistake, I can tell you in advance, was to entrust himself to the "gasoline" of carbohydrates, which he consumed all the time.

I don't know where the bizarre concept that "you have to eat several times a day to keep your metabolism active" came from. Who the heck said that? Nobody has been able to prove it. In terms of physiology or biochemistry, it is simply impossible. Bear that in mind, and if you do it yourself, it's time to reconsider. I myself followed that regime, I was taught that it was the right one, but it was a mistake. Now I know. I had to learn to unlearn in order to relearn.

So, if our diet is full of refined carbohydrates, fruit juices, processed foods, hydrogenated fats, and cheap, omega 6-rich oils, as the dietary systems we have almost everywhere in the world impose on us, we will keep inflaming our body and, despite our best efforts at the gym, on the street, on footpaths and athletics tracks, nothing will free us from a metabolic tragedy.

In recent years, the fitness trend has spread across the planet. And many enthusiasts started to believe that, in order to be super-healthy, they basically needed to nourish themselves with what was provided to them in a bunch of small containers. That's why they buy amino acids in a jar, proteins in a bottle, and everything promises to "taste like tropical pineapple from the Bahamas". It doesn't sound bad. And it doesn't taste good, because all of those little bottled wonders contain artificial flavors, colors and sweeteners. It's all artificial! But loads of people buy them because, as they are only thinking about "burning" and counting calories, those little pots are ideal because they don't contain any.

Maybe within they hold some hidden magic that the majority of us mere mortals just don't understand.

We need to stop this sick search for what appears to be something, but isn't. Maybe you're looking for the shake which tastes, looks and smells like chocolate, but isn't chocolate; what's more it's sweet, but doesn't contain any sugar; and, oh joy of joys, it's zero CAL! These sorts of products, for someone such as yourself on a personal crusade against the calorie monster, are a priceless discovery. The great global industry has made sure of that. Today we have many sweeteners like aspartame, maltodextrin, erythritol, sucralose, acesulfame K, neotame, saccharin or xylitol; we have a bunch of "sugars" which, in theory, as they contain no calories, are a wonder. However, I'd recommend you think about it more thoroughly. Why does it taste and smell like chocolate if it's not chocolate? Why is it sweet if it doesn't contain sugar? It is, but it isn't. Well, if what you want is to consume calorie-free chemicals, let's toast with a glass of Raid —zero calories—, a bar of soap —not a single calorie—, a glass of glyphosate herbicide or a shot of Dettol. It might sound over the top, but think about it.

Our body won't be better if we count calories or if we sweat our guts out with exercise and then don't eat well. And it won't feel more comfortable if we consume a diet high in little bottles or chemicals which replace real flavors and products. Nor will it if we think that the problem lies in our lack of will power to resist the "temptation" to eat. Maybe we don't have that will power because something is failing inside us. We talked about it a few pages ago. And here I must ask you to forget that belief —strengthened by the habits which our adorable grandmas and Aunt Bertha instilled in us— that "if my body asks me to, I must eat". Many patients tell me: "Doctor, my body is asking me for a slice of chocolate cake... Doctor, my body asks me for Coca-Cola at night... Doctor, the fridge talks to me!". Believe me, your body is not asking you for any of that. Metabolic problems, like obesity or diabetes, among others, are to do with a hormonal imbalance. And it's not about eating less, it's about eating better.

We forget that every meal is a choice and with every choice we make we are deciding what type of information we will give our organism. With each bite we are choosing between healing or sickness. There's no grey area. Each meal is decisive. What information will you give your body today? Bahamas tropical pineapple flavor? Are you going to keep counting calories after everything we have said in this chapter? Tell me you won't. Say it out loud.

Chapter 3

What makes us sick

If, after all, battling against those diabolical calories doesn't help to avoid obesity, if running like Forrest Gump and subjecting ourselves to a diet of two lettuce leaves a day does nothing to help us drop a few pounds, what's going wrong? What can we do?

Let's talk once and for all about those hormones. I'm going to try to explain it in the simplest possible way, so if there are any doctors present, welcome to *Sesame Street*. The first hormone on the list, the one I call the "queen" of our metabolic alterations, is insulin. This is produced in the pancreas and its main function is to regulate the behavior of the glucose in our body after we eat something. Food enters through the mouth, continues along down the esophagus, arrives at the stomach, passes into the small intestine, which takes charge of absorbing anything that is of use to our organism, in order to then permit its access to the blood stream; it then continues to the liver. Once it enters the blood, our body's "alarms" go off, the pancreas receives the alert and informs its pancreatic armed forces: "Hey, glucose (or carbohydrates or food) has just arrived", and it then produces insulin. This has two functions. On the one hand, it takes the glucose molecules, which is what provides energy to the cells, and sends 80 % of them to the organs that need it. On the other hand, it keeps some reserves and stores the remaining 20 % of glucose, which is converted into glycogen (its storage state) in the liver. And that excess, what's left over, is exported and stored in the fat, in the form of energy, to be used later. Said fat could be stored in the organs or the tissue under the skin. Those, in general terms, are the workings of our queen.

But insulin is like jealousy in a relationship: a little bit is fine, but an excess will cause enormous damage. When her Majesty —who is very important and necessary— is at the right levels, she will help our body to function in the ideal manner, although there are some professionals who don't pay any attention to this extremely important hormone. In fact, a few months ago a famous endocrinologist claimed on her social media accounts that doctors who order insulin tests to diagnose metabolic disorders should burn in hell because, she said, knowing the levels of that hormone is useless. I beg to differ, of course. And I invite you to burn in the fires of hell with me, through the pages of this book, in which the queen plays a starring role.

Almost always, when reference is made to insulin it is to remind us about that epidemic which has spread across the world, but to which we pay little attention despite there being new announcements on it almost daily; I'm talking about diabetes. Remember that this disease, which has quintupled globally in the last fifty years, has different forms. Type 1 diabetes is an autoimmune disease where the pancreas is unable to produce insulin: the glucose which the affected person ingests does not receive any help or guidance to find the right organs, or the liver, or wherever it should go and be of use. The glucose level in the blood will therefore be elevated and will produce different affectations, unless the insulin is injected into the body. Otherwise the person will die. But this specific illness affects less than 5 % of the planet's population. There is also the so-called type 1.5 diabetes —or adult type 1 diabetes (LADA)—, which at the end of the day behaves like what we have just described.

The one which affects the vast majority of the world's inhabitants is type 2. We used to call it "adult onset diabetes", but today we can't really use that term as there are patients aged 6 or 8 who suffer from it; I have had them in my practice. What causes it? An excess of insulin in the body.

The odd thing about it is that some specialists believe that the excess of this queen in our organism could be positive. There are even some medications used by endocrinologists for the treatment of diabetes and obesity which aim to stimulate the pancreas to produce more insulin. If we analyze this, it sounds fairly logical. 1) The patient has high blood sugar levels; 2) if there is a hormone to help remove this glucose from the blood stream, well the ideal thing to do would be to produce more of it; 3) unfortunately this reasoning takes us back to the example I gave you at the beginning of *The metabolic miracle*, when we talked about solving our flooded floor at home with an army of men with loads of mops. We're sticking with the consequences, and not examining the causes. At the end of the day, what will happen in the face of this excess of insulin is that the cell will fill up with glucose, exceed its tolerance limit, won't have space to store more, and part of it will be left outside the cell. And that is exactly how insulin resistance begins and the terrible onset of type 2 diabetes takes place.

It's like when you go on vacation and you're told you can only take one suitcase. It has a limit. If you try to pack too many things, they won't fit. You won't be able to close it, even if your whole family, including the heavyset Aunt Bertha, lies on top of it. When it doesn't fit, well, it doesn't fit. There are limits. That's life. And the same happens with our organism.

When the insulin arrives at the cell with the molecule of gluco-se, it will encounter a "doorman", the receptor; this will either say: "Yes ma'am, come on in" or "I'm sorry, there's no more space, go somewhere else". And trust me, in terms of the functioning of our metabolism, the old " Don't you know who I am? Open the door!" trick doesn't work. If the receptor puts up a blockade it's not for some alien reason, it does so because the cell no longer has space to put up its sweet guest. That is what resistance to insulin is, and it happens both within and outside the liver. And so where will the glucose go? The excess and a fraction of that which arrived direc-tly will end up in the liver. There it will turn into fat and yes, this is the start of the renowned fatty liver which, as you are beginning to realize, is not caused by the consumption of the macronutrient known as fat, but by the overabundance of carbohydrates and su-gars in our diet.

When the liver can't store any more glucose, it will produce fat. This will build up between the cells and not inside them. Fatty liver leads to non-alcoholic fatty liver disease, which has seen an enormous increase across the globe, well above the rate of alco-holic cirrhosis. And it all began because the body started to create more insulin than it should.

Insulin is guilty of causing various disorders in our organism, which is why it is necessary to have it under control. Every day I see to more patients with obesity and metabolic disorders, eleva-ted triglycerides and fatty liver, who have been given as a solution a good dosage of pills to lower cholesterol and triglycerides. I'm sorry, that is not the way out. The root of the problem is not being studied. High triglycerides are also the result of an excess of car-bohydrates (the bad ones), because these are what unsettle Her Majesty, insulin.

Frequently, when specialists want to examine their patients' metabolism, the only thing they prescribe is a lipid panel, a gly-caemia test on an empty stomach and a thyroid examination. End of story. It is always recommendable to check the glucose (sugar) and insulin (the hormone which regulates it) levels dynamically, that is to say by following the behavior of both of them after stimulating them and after eating. Among these two measurements we can find "clinical gems" which will make all the difference.

I suppose you have had a pre and post meal glycaemia test. The first measurement is taken of the glycemic levels on an empty stomach; the second, after the patient has taken a load of glucose —anguish for some— and waiting two hours to see how the body behaves in the face of this ingestion. And here's another interesting detail: one piece of evidence that suggests you may have high insulin levels is that your post-meal glycaemia results (the second test) are lower than the pre-meal results. How can that happen? It sounds illogical, I know, but if your metabolism is disrupted and it produces more insulin, well the insulin will be responsible for evacuating all that sugar you consumed from the blood and, due to an abundance of the queen hormone, at the end of the test you will have less glucose than at the beginning. This is called "high insulin sensitivity", which indicates that your body still adapts to the elevated dosage and activity of insulin.

It is often believed that this behavior is normal just because the results fall within permitted value ranges, but if a patient has 80 mg/dL (milligrams per deciliter) on an empty stomach, and after receiving a load of glucose shows 70 mg/dL, that is an indication that should be taken into account. Why? Imagine that you arrive at the gas station with your tank almost empty. As you're going on a trip you decided to fill up. However, two hours later the fuel gauge tells you that you only have a quarter of a tank left. You will immediately assume that something is wrong with your car's engine. If your post-meal glycaemia test shows lower levels than your pre-meal test, perhaps you should be thinking the same thing. It's likely that something is up with your metabolism.

This is the initial phenomenon. I see it a lot in children and adolescents. Doctors check these tests and tell them they have hypoglycemia, so the solution, they say, is for them to eat every three hours to fix it and ideally, they tell the parents, the kid should eat something sweet. Is that the best option? No. That will just make everything worse.

What will happen is that, as the patient has produced so much insulin —because this gets going every time the person eats—, their cells will fill up with glucose until the doorman says: "Look for somewhere else to stay". The blood tests will quickly show what happened. Maybe the glycaemia levels in this patient on an empty stomach (pre-meal) are at 80 mg/dL. Then they ingest the load of glucose and the results will change significantly. The expected measurement in any person with a regular metabolism should show an increase of 10 to 15 units, around 90 or 95 mg/dL, which will indicate that two hours after ingesting the glucose, the organism was able to store some of this in the cells and a little extra was left over unabsorbed, to be consumed later. It's normal. But if the results show measurements of 120 or 130 mg/dL, for example, that's proof that the organism could not store the glucose in the cells. There wasn't enough space. They were full of sugar. This is clear evidence of insulin resistance, the cause of type 2 diabetes, which afflicts 95 % of the world's diabetics and which is causing cardiovascular and metabolic diseases, and strokes, among other afflictions.

Insulin resistance causes, in some cases, chronic high cholesterol; it produces, in all cases, elevated triglycerides; it causes increased obesity and adiposity, and is also guilty of a heap of infertility problems, because it causes polycystic ovaries. Although women are often told the opposite: "Miss, your polycystic ovaries generate insulin resistance". No. It's the other way around, doctor. They are the result of an excess of production of the queen, which eventually alters the physiology of the hormones, which in turn unsettles the ovary and it all turns into a vicious cycle.

But the origin of the problem lies in the pancreas, the gland which produces insulin, and which was altered by an unsuitable dietary model (it all starts with that simple act). The queen will not only contribute to creating cysts in the ovaries; she will also cause terminated pregnancies. Many women won't manage to give birth. After seven or eight weeks their bodies cannot continue with the gestation because the elevated insulin competes with the progesterone, the hormone which allows the pregnancy to follow its course.

Insulin, friend or foe?

Recent studies show that one in three people on the planet has prediabetes in one of its forms. Relax, that doesn't mean that 33.3 % of humanity is on the verge of diabetes. What the studies show is that this is the percentage of patients who already have at least one test showing disrupted glucose and insulin levels. They are simply warning signs that remind us that this reality can be altered with better eating habits.

I want to reiterate, regardless of if I will burn in hell, as that celebrity endocrinologist claims, that insulin is a hormone which we must check and measure dynamically. The glucose test is not enough; we have to examine this hormone in the same way, on an empty stomach and after eating. If for some reason you couldn't obtain that measurement, al least ask for a dynamic glucose test. If you see alterations, I suggest you use the old adage " If you think the worst, you will not be far wrong"; it's highly likely that your insulin is disrupted. Taking care of it will bring you great benefits.

Knowing how under control the queen is has a trick to it. I tend to see a lot of cases of patients with normal glycaemia levels but disrupted insulin levels. We need to be careful and demand this test!

What are the parameters for knowing if our insulin levels are within the acceptable range? In my patients, I look for readings of under 5 uIU/ml on an empty stomach and under 30 uIU/ml after a glucose load. Other specialists are laxer with their ranges. It's worth noting that the reference values at most laboratories are very permissive and do not help the doctor to identify when the results are bad. What is within normal limits for them is sometimes a sign of diabetes for me.

Don't forget that this illness is not a problem caused by high blood sugar levels. That is the consequence. Diabetes is produced because we have a disorder in our insulin metabolism. Due to this disorder, it's just the same having it without it being able to do its job, as it is not having it. In conclusion, we should always request both tests: glycaemia and insulin; they will give us clearer clues about the health of those we are trying to care for.

I persevere with this because, beyond the Functional Medicine theories, which many doctors look down on, my experience has shown me that those patients who I have helped to correct their insulin levels have started to show improvements in their cholesterol, triglyceride and sugar levels; they start to lose weight, their acne subsides, women get their menstruation back; and those who couldn't get pregnant manage to do so. It's not the consequence of some miracle. It's not the fruit of my "superpowers". It is the result of a long process of studies, reading, and delving deeper into the understanding of biochemistry and nutritional biochemistry. That is how I have managed to guide my patients better and encourage them to obtain these positive results. So let there be no doubt: insulin, the queen of the hormones, performs a starring role in the majority of metabolic problems on the planet —hell, here I come—.

Remember that food is the most valuable information that we give our organism, because, among other things, food positively or negatively affects the hormones which control our metabolism. Of the three macronutrients which we will talk about in this book: carbohydrates, proteins and fats, the former are the ones which most stimulate insulin production. But each carbohydrate has a different effect on insulin; you can't compare the effect of broccoli —remember that vegetables are carbohydrates— to that which can be caused by some cookies with artificial vanilla cream, some sugary candy or several shots of *aguardiente*. Each one provokes a different spike in this hormone.

Second, we have proteins. Of course they also stimulate insulin. Surprised? Of course, nobody tells you that. You may well have started a high protein diet —they are all the rage— and you're feeling very proud of that, because those good girls don't have a glycemic index and that's why they come so highly recommended! And it's obvious: only glucose has one. A piece of steak is sugar-free. But be careful not to surpass the limit, because an excess of protein also converts into glucose. We can store a bit of this in the liver, as glycogen; but when this organ can no longer absorb any more of it, it converts it into fat. Yes, you're reading this right; just as we said a few lines ago, glucose ends up transforming into fat. That is what our body does in order to store energy coming from food, which can be used in moments when we have no food available.

Of the three macronutrients, it's the healthy fats which stimulate insulin the least. There are debates on the topic. Various authors state that they cause no stimulation to the queen whatsoever; but they do, very subtly perhaps, but they do affect her. That's why, if our diet includes a high percentage of healthy fats and good carbohydrates —vegetables mainly—, we will produce less insulin and will also be able to control our metabolism more easily.

This dear hormone is directly related to the number of kilos we gain or lose. That is evident in those patients who are slightly overweight and, as a result of their poor eating habits, start to develop type 2 diabetes due to insulin resistance. Many of them are given insulin injections. If you have been paying attention to what I have explained in this section, you will understand that this is the same as using the well-known clothing vacuum bags to try to get more clothing, or whatever it may be, into that travel suitcase which is already full. And again, the whole family and heavy Aunt Bertha will jump up and down on the suitcase to try to close it. But it's on the verge of bursting! This is the same effect on the body that will be experienced by those who have developed a resistance to insulin and also receive the injections. If the patient previously underwent oral treatment with, for example, metformin, but they are told they need to receive insulin injections, they will start to gain weight in a drastic fashion. It doesn't fail. Just as they begin the treatment, they pile on the pounds. Strange, right?

Well, not really. There's nothing strange about it. It's a fact. This hormone is responsible for us gaining weight, having metabolic syndrome, developing diabetes, having increased triglycerides and cholesterol, and for cardiovascular diseases and strokes arising more frequently. How do we avoid all this? How do we control it? With thousands of pills and injections? No. It's easy: by eating right.

Leptin, faithful friend

However, metabolism doesn't just depend on insulin. In many cases, we work hard with our patients to control it and, after some time, what a surprise! The imbalances persist. It's then that we have to check on the queen's group of "buddies". One of this gang's major players is a hormone called leptin.

It is produced in fat cells, which we also call the adipose tissue or adipocyte. What is its purpose? The main one is sending a signal to the brain, which says: "Hey, we're satisfied, there's no room for more food". When that happens, we feel full. "Really, doctor, that's what this leptin does? And that's important?", you'll be asking me. Of course it is. We humans are the only mammal, the only animal on the planet, which eats out of greed; oh! And we are the only obese species on the planet —a terrifying fact. Only we, out of anxiety, end up eating everything that we shouldn't—. Yes, researchers can induce a mouse to eat out of anxiety, that's true, but we will talk about that in the chapter on sugar. If leptin didn't exist, we might eat until we explode, much like Mr. Creosote, the incredibly fat character from Monty Python's *The Meaning of Life*.

Luckily leptin exists. It was discovered not long ago, in 1994, by Dr. Jeffrey M. Friedman and his team. This revelation immediately became a source of joy for many people. They thought that, with this finding, the cure for obesity had arrived, because, if we could control leptin levels, compulsive eaters would be able to keep their mouths shut. That's us, always looking for easy fixes to problems which require another kind of solution. But I'm not going to make a detailed analysis of this hormone, I just wanted to introduce it to you so that you keep it in mind. So that you remember it every time you put your hand on your stomach and say: "I'm full!".

When we study cases of people suffering obesity, diabetes or metabolic problems, we end up discovering that they have high leptin levels. And this reached such levels because insulin levels were also elevated. Just as there is a resistance to the latter, as we have seen, our body will also develop resistance to the former. In many cases, this point is reached because the patient has put themselves in the hands of those specialists or industries who claim to work on the "obesity gene". But, just so that we are speaking the same language, this gene, although it exists, has not shown any clinical benefits. What these doctors do is to create treatments to stimulate leptin. And, as with almost all of these procedures, their way of working sounds logical. If there is a patient who eats too much and wants to leave obesity behind, well it would be a good idea for them to have more leptin, which is the hormone screaming: "I'm stuffed, I can't eat any more". But, what seems logical ends up causing a metabolic disorder. Hence, just like what happens with insulin, the body develops a resistance to leptin. And the patient will get fatter. They will reach the worst case scenario, saying: "Doctor, I eat and I eat and I never feel full". Their metabolism is so out of whack that it doesn't know how interpret the "stop, don't eat any more" signals. **The brain stops understanding reason. It doesn't understand anything. How did it get to that point? High insulin levels, high leptin levels. Wrong treatment, metabolic disorder.** And there is a poison, which we will soon discover, and which makes an immense contribution to this tragedy because it has a secret weapon: although it enters our organism, it never stimulates leptin. It goes by unnoticed. All clear up until now?

TEST
HOW ARE YOU FEELING TODAY?

Before continuing on this hormonal journey, please answer this new questionnaire as honestly as possible. You already know the methodology. Just answer *Yes* or *No*.

	YES	NO
Do you feel tired during the day?		
Have you lost interest in things that previously gave you pleasure?		
Do you wake up full of energy between 1:00 and 3:00 in the morning and then find it hard to get back to sleep?		
Have you had a recent drop in your sex drive?		
After exercising, is your recovery slow?		
Do you experience tachycardia or heart palpitations after making slight exertions?		
Are you experiencing a decrease in your memory, the capacity to learn and perform your job or daily tasks normally?		
Have you recently been ill more than usual?		
Have you experienced an unexplained amount of hair loss recently?		
Do you feel like your mind is "foggy"?		

Have you recently been in a "flat" mood?		
Do you experience frequent teeth grinding or muscular pain?		
Do you feel drowsiness during the day?		

If you responded in the affirmative to several of these questions, I suggest that you read the next section carefully. Let me introduce you to your good friend cortisol; maybe he is trying to tell you something.

Cortisol the courtier

Cortisol is also part of Queen Insulin's court and is very important. It is produced in the adrenal glands, located above the kidneys. Cortisol is the lead guitarist of the "band" of steroid hormones which stem from cholesterol, such as testosterone, estrogen and progesterone —the male and female sexual hormones—, but also fronts the group which plays with our sympathetic nervous system, which is responsible for activating our body's response to threats or stress.

Cortisol interacts with almost all of our organs. Thanks to cortisol, we can adapt to life's worries: the stress of existence and facing a new day, stress caused by traffic, thermal stress cause by heat, emotional stress, the stress of illness or a chronic or painful infection. Cortisol is what allows us to activate that valuable *fight or flight* mechanism when faced with danger.

Let me explain: if you have been through states of anxiety, if you have suffered from panic attacks or depression, your psychologist or psychiatrist will no doubt have spoken to you about it, about how, thousands of years ago, when our ancestors were faced with the presence of a ferocious beast, they felt a state of alarm which allowed them to react and save their lives. And it is still very effective.

These days, we don't have to deal with saber-toothed tigers every day, but we do face other dangers linked to our lifestyle. I'm talking about poor diets, lack of sleep and exercise, the effects of radiation or various chemicals, pollution or cigarette smoke; and also our own shortfalls, lack of acceptance, low self-esteem, copying external models, wanting to live the life that those "happy kids" publish on Instagram. All of that provokes stress, and so it stimulates the production of this good friend of Queen Insulin.

I like to explain that cortisol should work like when we charge our cellphone battery. I leave mine charging every night so that, at 5:00 in the morning, the battery is ready to be used throughout the day without any problems. That's how our cortisol should work. Ideally, in the morning it should be completely available for use throughout the day and at night it should be able to go to bed. You may not know this, but our body's hormones have different timetables, some of them work the day shift and others take the night shift. Cortisol is an employee who is more productive in the first shift; if the poor guy ends up working overtime, we're going to have a problem.

Going back to the cellphone analogy, if I want to use it at 2:00 in the morning and interrupt its charging, it's likely that at about 6:00 my phone will only have about 70 % of the battery available and will stop working at midday, in the middle of an important conversation. What will I do then? Charge it in the late afternoon or early evening. So I will always have high battery levels at the least favorable times, and at the most important times my cellphone will stop working. Is it the phone's fault? No, it's my fault for following a bad timetable.

That's what tends to happen to the cortisol in many of my patients. They wake up in the morning with low levels —that is to say, with the battery at 50 or 60 %— and they feel tired for the whole day. But their cortisol keeps on "charging" and reaches full battery at times when they should be sleeping, let's say at 1:00 or 2:00 in the morning. I tend to ask them: "Are you often awake at those hours? And if so, if you had to get up at that time of the night and take the dog for a walk or do your supermarket shop, could you do that?". They all respond: "Yes, doctor, of course! Not just that, I could run a half marathon at 2:00 in the morning". Their cortisol is reaching its maximum levels at the wrong times! And, what's more, they lie awake, clearheaded, all night. On the edge of sleepwalking, those patients might manage to sleep a bit more during the night, but the next day they wake up as if they have been run over by a steamroller. And, take a note of this, elevated cortisol levels raise insulin levels. These two buddies will have a party which will always cause a metabolic imbalance.

I want to give you one more fact about the hormonal "shifts". Cortisol, under normal circumstances, should be working very actively during the day; let's say it prefers normal office hours. But if its work day is extended or it starts its shift between 1:00 and 3:00 in the morning, Houston, we have a problem! At those hours, the liver should come into action, as it works best in the early hours. So what happens? Well, the cortisol takes the shift allotted to that organ, causing deficiencies in its detoxification process and causing an increase in its consumption of glycogen at night, which in turn will produce elevated glycaemia levels in the morning. This is known as elevated nocturnal glycogenolysis (the breakdown or use of liver glycogen at night).

Imbalances caused by cortisol affect millions of people around the world and can turn into the erroneously named "chronic fatigue" or "adrenal fatigue". I say erroneously named because the term is, in effect, incorrect. It is the imbalance of the hypothalamic-pituitary-adrenal axis, which refers to the route taken by cortisol, from the brain (hypothalamus and pituitary gland) to its final production in the adrenal gland.

These imbalances also cause fibromyalgia, memory loss in young people, chronic sleep disturbances, loss of sex drive, chronic tiredness during the day, loss of interest in activities that were previously enjoyed, depressive moods or even depression per se; as well as poor adaptation to exercise, poor recovery from trauma and repeated viral or bacterial infections (due to low defenses). All of these symptoms need to be evaluated, analyzed and treated by a specialist in the topic —ideally a Functional Medicine expert—. The signs I just mentioned will mean that our metabolism will be in turmoil in every sense, from the production of insulin to the production of triglycerides and cholesterol.

When the queen and her neighborhood chum get together a warning signal goes off, because the greater the amount of cortisol —or the greater the imbalance in its normal functioning— the greater the production of insulin. As we already mentioned, when this increases, metabolic problems and inflammation are generated, and the body gets stressed. And what happens if the organism is stressed? Well, it will produce more cortisol. More cortisol... more insulin. This creates a vicious cycle.

This behavior is typical in those patients who, due to the diseases they suffer from, are injected with or administered medications derived from or similar to cortisol, such as the infamous corticosteroids. These always lead to a weight increase in people. Why do they put on weight? Because they end up increasing their glucose, and therefore their insulin. Corticosteroids are everywhere, doctors recommend them for treating asthmatic children —inhaled—, for dermatological problems —applied to the skin— and for other respiratory disorders because they are very good anti-inflammatories —orally—.

We said that cortisol helps us with stress, but our body is not prepared to put up with the chronic stress we live with at all times these days. The overwhelming and permanent presence of stress causes our organism to fail. It's like when an empty glass starts to receive a drop of water every hour. For a long time, it can hold, without any trouble, that small amount which falls into it. Over the days —or months, depending on its size— the water will begin to fill the glass and it will spill. Thus, the drop which previously caused absolutely no trauma will now cause a disaster. The liquid overflows. The same thing happens with chronic stress.

Numerous patients have told me: "But, doctor, for the last 10 years I have always lived with these stress levels. I have always worked under pressure and responded well. I don't know why I have broken down now, if nothing has changed". Yes, something did change, the last drop arrived, which made the glass overflow. Their body couldn't take any more. The cortisol fought as best it could. It did well for a very long time. It was overworked for years. And, worse still, it got together with its friend, insulin. So this unsettled their metabolism. The desperate cycle we already mentioned began. And thus the so-called general adaptation syndrome was provoked. It happened because the cortisol covered a shift that wasn't his. This can all result in an extreme state, something strange, which is chronic fatigue, which is produced when there is very low or inexistent cortisol throughout the day, and is the result of various metabolic failures in our body. It is a very uncommon occurrence.

If you're reading these lines and notice that something similar happens to you, no doubt you will want to ask your general practitioner to refer you to get your cortisol levels checked. Why not? But be aware that the majority of professionals will order a blood test to take this measurement; however, clinically, said test will be of no use. The cortisol test should be a saliva test. (Today, dry urine tests, which are a very efficient way to measure it, are also carried out, but they are only available in the United States). In any case it will require the analysis of a specialist who knows the physiological metabolism of cortisol as a hormone off by heart —as well as its role within the hormonal system itself and the nervous system—.

One test is not enough. Cortisol is an elusive fellow. Sometimes we carry out the test and find high levels in a patient who should have low levels, or vice versa. That's why there needs to be a very detailed monitoring process, because maybe our patient had high levels in the early morning —the unexpected hours— and low levels during the day. In order to ensure we are not mistaken, as doctors we need to understand this hormone very well, understand how it can be altered due to our modern lifestyle, how we are going to diagnose it and how we are going to treat it. And we should know that, if it is disrupted, that it because it has also begun to play inappropriate games with other "friends". Cortisol is like a rebellious teenager who just wants to be understood.

Uric acid

Now I'm going to introduce you to the fourth squire of this royal court, made up of the hormones insulin (produced by the pancreas and captain of glucose), leptin (produced in fat cells and commander of feeling full) and cortisol (produced by the adrenal gland and admiral of stress). The other member is uric acid. This is a waste product formed in all the body's cells as part of the elimination of deoxyribonucleic acid (more popularly known as DNA), which is housed inside the cell's nucleus. It is an organic, natural compound and appropriate for when the cells are renewing. During this process our DNA will break up and reconfigure, which is why it needs to leave the cells so that it can be eliminated through the kidneys.

Why do uric acid levels rise? For two main reasons: because our body produces a lot or because we eliminate too little. Which illness recurs when the levels are elevated? We always think of gout, a form of arthritis which manifests itself as pain in the big toe, the knees or the elbows, or which can even cause bodily deformities —large nodules called *tophi*—. Some people present these symptoms as a result of high consumption of red meat, pork, cold cuts or red wine, but gout is not the only illness that our new neighborhood pal produces. In fact, it is even one of the least common.

First we need to understand something: within the cell and at normal levels, uric acid has protective, antioxidant qualities. It does valuable work. But if there is too much of it in our body, it will remain outside the cell and have toxic effects, cause inflammation in our organism and lead to illness. And what can make the uric acid levels rise? There is a quick route, known as the fructan pathway, meaning an excess of the infamous fructose in our diet will cause the rise. We will have long discussions about this fruit sugar in the coming chapters. For now, just remember that it is a uric acid enhancer.

Ok. If we have an excess of fructose in the body, one of the biggest fools will be the liver, who will think that it is "raining" fructose inside itself and will start to produce a lot of uric acid in response to this sugary rain. Due to the amount of energy required to carry out this process and the degradation of the energy units known as ATP, these will end up producing extremely high levels of uric acid.

Such an increase has the potential to raise the insulin and cortisol levels, and as we've already seen, it is best to keep this couple apart. But it's not just that: with uric acid levels through the roof, the organism will begin to cancel the production of nitric oxide, which carries out a crucial role, ensuring our arteries are dilated so that the blood can flow through them without any issues. If there is too little nitric oxide, the arteries will be tense and this could lead to arterial hypertension, a very frequent and recurrent cause of high blood pressure. So, the excess of uric acid does not only cause a metabolic disorder: it can turn into a cardiovascular risk factor.

Summing up, how did this all come to happen? So much fructose forces the liver to work more; it also provokes a rise in uric acid levels, and this stimulates the cortisol, which in turn will affect the insulin via multiple pathways. Another dangerous cycle, this time with more cast members.

If our organism gets used to an excess of fructose, a slight stimulus will be enough for it to flick its internal switch and contribute to metabolic disorder. When we follow a diet which is high in fructans, for example, we are helping keep the switch on. What are fructans? They are found in onions, garlic, asparagus, apples, pears, peaches, grapes, mangoes, watermelons, almonds, pistachios, fermented foods, beer, red beans and white cheeses, among other products. Some of you will be saying: "What do you mean, doctor? Garlic does more good than Pope Francis!". Yes, of course, garlic has wonderful anti-inflammatory properties, helps against infections and even against cancer. It may well be very good for all human beings, but *not* at every moment in life. If we have become accustomed to a dietary regime with an abundance of fructose, when we receive a fructan like garlic we might flick that internal switch I was telling you about.

That's why it is so important to stop thinking that gout is the only illness related to high levels of uric acid. Doctors, in general, pay very little attention to this "little friend" of insulin and cortisol, but it should never be dismissed. I recommend the uric acid measurement test to the majority of my patients with metabolic problems and the results almost always surprise us. The levels are high and that was the last thing they expected. Why? As I said at the outset, specialists think that this check is unnecessary because the person who walked into their practice didn't show symptoms of gout. Today, it is hugely important to run the test and understand the workings of uric acid. And it's worth revising the reference values we still use when looking at the results. Recent studies show that the levels in women should be below 4 mg/dL and below 5.5 mg/dL in men. The numerical limits which the laboratories use tend to be well above these ranges because they are reporting results with gout in mind, and usually they only consider levels above 7 mg/dL to be high.

One moment, and what about the thyroid?

When I started working on this book, I asked myself that question many times. The thyroid is an extremely important gland, located at the base of the neck, just in front of the trachea, which produces the thyroid hormones, to which all of the body's cell have to respond; it is also an important metabolic commander.

One of my main jobs as a doctor is to guarantee my patients that their thyroid gland is working correctly. If any of them shows abnormalities, we work in detail in order to understand the causes of the variation, until we can correct it. In functional medicine we don't have a set formula or prescription for all of our patients, we don't prescribe levothyroxine to everyone —as is the norm— in order to begin the game of increasing or decreasing the dosage depending on the elevation or reduction of the TSH (thyroid-stimulating hormone) values.

There are a lot of possible things which might affect thyroid functioning: raised cortisol levels due to stress, chronic infections, nutrient deficiencies... That's why I repeat that each case must be checked in isolation in order to find the real cause of the alteration. The thyroid, alone, deserves an entire book, and going into details on it would sidetrack us from the main point of *The metabolic miracle*. The main thing is this: in the case of a thyroid disorder, we need to know what caused it. It needs to work well.

I am going to end this chapter by mentioning some hormones that are also relevant to our metabolism and whose existence we should know about, like ghrelin (related to our appetite), adiponectin (produced by the adipose tissue), peptide YY (a neurotransmitter with a hormonal response behavior) and cholecystokinin (produced in the small intestine). This group make up the supporting actors of this metabolic movie, starring our queen, insulin and her band of buddies, cortisol, leptin and uric acid. Understanding their behavior is essential to taking the correct steps in combating metabolic syndrome diseases around the world.

And why haven't they told me that?

I don't want to move on to the next chapter without first trying to answer some other doubts that I know you must have. I've called for you to be more alert to your insulin levels, I've introduced some hormones that perhaps weren't of interest to you, I've told you that healthy fats don't clog arteries, and that calorie counting doesn't work, and I've constantly repeated the fact that each mouthful is information for the body, among other statements. It's very likely that you've never heard your family physician talk about any of this. So you'd be justified in showing some mistrust and doubt. **You'll wonder: "Why did my doctor, who knows me, and who has treated me forever, not tell me about these things? Why change my routines and take the plunge into terra incognita? Why do my family doctors tell me that this Functional Medicine doesn't exist and that it is a 21st century scam? Does this Doctor Jaramillo know what he's talking about? Is he** a heretic? What must the poor man eat?". Doubts are welcome, questions are welcome. *If I were a reader of* The metabolic miracle, *I too would have my qualms.* But each line that I write has scientific backing and is supported by my years of study and work with patients; years of learning, practicing, observing and results.

It turns out that when we take different approaches to the traditional ones, to the approved, learnt and unrefuted truth, doctors —"colleagues"— immediately come out to discredit us, to shout: "Show me the evidence, where is it? Show it to me, show it to me!". That which is pointed to as false and absurd today, will no longer be seen that way tomorrow if a study appears which legitimizes it. That means that the thing which was criticized was neither false nor absurd, just that at the time not all the required evidence existed. Or that, despite it existing, there was little political will or real interest from the various players (the pharmaceutical industry, different brands, academia itself, among others) to bring it to light.

But medicine can't work like this. We need to practice with bravery —without being reckless— and understand that the body's greatest wealth of evidence can be found with a deeper understanding of physiology, biochemistry and immunology. Only thus can we debate new findings, even if they are recently published.

I'd like to highlight a phrase I heard from the wise British professor and writer Sir Ken Robinson —you may have heard one of his conferences on the global educational model—: "If you're not prepared to be wrong, you'll never come up with anything original". It is important to remove our fear of failing. Nobody is infallible. But always following the safe route will not help us to learn and find new solutions. To those who walk into my practice, I often say: "I don't know the cause of your illness yet, but together we will find it".

There are two types of doctor: 1) those who just read or carry out studies, and 2) those who see to patients and understand that a lot of the scientific evidence does not fit the reality of the

people we are trying to heal, and who also realize that nothing has been written about many of the things we see on a daily basis. And that does not mean that the evidence does not exist, it's there and it's real, but perhaps the study backing it up has not yet been written.

I'll give you an example of what I am saying: the emotional factors which impact patients suffering from obesity will never make up part of a scientific analysis of the topic. But I see them all the time in my practice and I handle them with those manifesting them. Because we mustn't forget that "the absence of evidence is not evidence of absence".

Going back to what we have seen in this chapter, someone might say that everything I have said about insulin is nonsense or heresy, and they might ask where the study which took into account at least 10,000 patients after measuring their hormone levels is. What is for sure is that I have treated thousands of them with the theories I have coined —product of my years of study, specialization and work— and every day they provide more evidence. If, in a few months, some organization manages to cure thousands of sick people with my "ridiculous and heretic" theories on, let's say, insulin, then they will say that everything has been proven; "that Jaramillo isn't as mad as he appeared; he wasn't a charlatan after all".

To conclude, I just want to remind you of two things. The first is that the evidence we have spoken about, evidence from the world of science, is supported by three fundamental pillars: 1) The best available evidence from scientific investigation; 2) the preferences of patients and respect for them and their values, and 3) the clinical experience of those carrying out the study and/or evaluating its findings. That was how Professor David Sackett, promoter of evidence-based medicine (EBM) proposed it. But these three components are not generally taken into account in a rigorous fashion. Usually, the "evidence" is gathered and presented by those who want to show that their product works (whether it's a food product, powdered Bahamas piña colada, or medication). Do you really think that the majority of companies on the planet would be willing to have it proven that one of their creations —with which they hope to rake in millions of dollars— doesn't do what it promises or that it causes problems to consumers? I doubt it. That's why the large soft drink companies who make "life taste good" are the ones who finance studies into artificial sweeteners and their benefits. That way they can prove that their inventions are good; they create the evidence —with their own pillars—.

And the second thing is that it has been shown that 50 % of the knowledge that all of us doctors acquire during our studies, and which we considered true and correct, will be re-evaluated or become evidence which doesn't contribute anything five years after we graduate, it's just that we don't know what that 50 % will be. That's why, as professionals, we don't have any other choice but to keep studying, keep learning and dedicating ourselves to reading, reading and reading. That process includes reading all authors, those who we admire and follow; and those who we do not agree with or don't have an affinity with, but who also contribute to the profession. We can't lose our curiosity or our interest, we must have the bravery and humility to unlearn a concept, learn a new one and understand how it will help us help the human being in front of us. This is Medicine's ultimate goal: to cure our patients.

So this book is, on the one hand, for those colleagues of mine who, distancing themselves from prejudice and mistrust, want to unlearn; for all those people who I have seen to in my practice and from whom I have learnt so much, and, of course, for you, the reader of *The metabolic miracle*, who in some ways I also consider my patient, because if you are reading these lines it is because you are looking for solutions which I hope to help you find.

Chapter 4

Anxiety and food addiction

In April 2007, in the English scientific journal *The Lancet*, Doctor David Nutt, professor at the Psychopharmacology Unit of the University of Bristol (United Kingdom), and three collaborators published an article about the 20 most dangerous and addictive substances in the world. They divided them into three categories, according to the harm they cause people, the dependence they generate and their effect on society. In the "dependency" category, the study took three parameters into account: the intensity of the pleasure offered by those substances, the psychological dependency and the physical dependency they create. On a scale of 0 to 3, with 0 meaning no risk; 1, some risk; 2, moderate risk, and 3, high risk, the most addictive substances in this score were heroin (3.0), cocaine (2.39), barbiturates (2.01) and, in fourth place, alcohol (1.93).

These results were shared in the world's most important media outlets and are still being quoted today. The investigation reminded us of some of our recurring weaknesses as human beings. We could add to this list, addictions to gambling, sex, pornography, videogames and social media; addictions which are also discussed in the news. But what really grabs my attention is that we don't place any importance on one of the major illnesses that we currently have on the planet: addiction to food, a problem which we still can't properly gauge.

We are on the brink of the third decade of the 21st century and most people don't know how and what to eat, or we don't understand why we are eating all day and, furthermore, why we want to do it continuously. Lurking behind all those unresolved questions is the worst counsellor of all, the world's massive food industry, which does tell us, with its advertising wisdom, what and how to eat. It bombards us with its commercials, promotions, prizes and suggestions. It yells to us: "Try this, there's no risk, it's fat-free, it uses an artificial sweetener and is low in calories; eat it, it's fantastic. It doesn't provide you with anything, but it tastes good". It constantly encourages us to make poor decisions.

On the road to addiction, sugar is the first signpost. It should have made up part of David Nutt's list. If his analysis shows that cocaine is the second most addictive substance in the world, with a score of 2.39 out of 3.0, we should then be much more careful with sugar (the poison of the West), because it causes more addiction than cocaine.

That's not just me saying it. It isn't part of my "heresy". It has been proven in studies of neuroimaging which have checked, in an active and dynamic fashion, the brain centers which control anxiety and people's addictions (the accumbens nucleus). These tests have proven that the stimulus produced by sugar in this region is eight times greater than that produced by cocaine. Eight times greater!

That's why I would dare to say that this little white friend which sweetens our life is even more addictive than heroin. "Show me

the evidence, doctor!", the choir of skeptics will cry. I am not aware of a list similar to that of Nutt which includes sugar. However, if
somebody were to try to carry out a similar study, it would be difficult to complete; the industry's large companies would impede
it at all costs. Yet, seen under the light of neuroimaging, the power
that sugar holds over us is devastating. I have seen what it does to
many of my patients.

It is often thought that people eat relentlessly because they are
"anxious"; however, it is the food which is causing them the anxiety. By picking the wrong foods, they are giving their body bad information and provoking a neuroendocrine abnormality. That is
to say that they stimulate their brain centers, and the notorious
hormones we spoke about in the previous chapter, in the wrong
way. If we excessively activate our insulin (which helps the glucose
enter our cells) and leptin (which gives the "I'm full" signal), chaos
will ensue and we will be hungry and anxious to keep eating the
whole time.

The contradictory thing is that, in such a case, eating is not
the solution, it is the act which intensifies the short circuit. It's
as if we have been possessed by a weird and powerful spirit
which does not stop repeating: "We have to eat, we have to
eat. More and more!". Unfortunately, when we are hungry, our
brain doesn't think: "How delicious a bit of broccoli with carrot
would be right now". Of course not. When our appetite is at
the ready, the spirit inside wants a piece of cake, bread with
jelly and a soft drink, chocolate cookies with vanilla cream. We
want something sweet, we crave sugar: adding fuel to the fire!
Get to work, Mrs. Insulin, Mr. Leptin and friends.

The sad thing is that our greed does not have that reward mechanism which our pets have. If our dog is anxious, we give him a
cookie and, lo and behold, he will likely calm down. Likewise, an
alcoholic will feel great satisfaction after having a drink, the same
satisfaction felt by a compulsive smoker upon taking a drag on

their obligatory post-coffee cigarette. The drink and the tobacco are their respective rewards. However, those who feel anxiety and addiction towards food will not receive any pleasure upon feeding themselves. This is proven. Satisfying their appetite generates guilt rather than pleasure. That is why eating disorders such as bulimia exist. If that guilt did not exist, people would not go to the bathroom to vomit after eating.

Let's now go back to the early 20th century. There, in his scientific bunker, sits Russian physiologist Ivan Petrovich Pavlov, who won the Nobel Prize in 1904 and became the father of classical conditioning. But before that happened, the good man worked with his dogs and other collaborators in the study which would later make him famous. He was trying to understand when and why those canines drooled. He noticed that they did it when they saw food. He then began to ring a bell before feeding them. With the passing of time, the dogs began to understand that, after it rang, they would eat, so they would start salivating. Days later, just the bell ringing —without the presence of food— would cause the dogs to drool. The doctor had provoked what is known as a conditioned response. If the bell rang, the saliva would start to spill out of the dogs' mouths. What does Pavlov have to do with our topic? Let me explain.

The Russian realized that, if the same stimulus was repeated for 21 days, he could create a conditioned response. We too have provoked dozens of them. The morning cigarette? The coffee and slice of cake just after lunch? The single malt on a Friday night? Sound familiar? Well, I don't know at what wretched moment we were told (or commanded) that we had to eat every two or three hours in order to "activate the metabolism" and so that the body "isn't left without energy" —I've said it before, I even believed it because the nutritionists recommended it—. It was a lie, of course. A lie that greatly pleased food producers because it meant that we would consume more of their products. So suddenly we began to eat breakfast at 7:00 in the morning, have a "bite" at 10:00, have lunch at 1:00 in the afternoon, eat a snack at 4:00, have dinner at 7:30 in the evening, and perhaps even force ourselves to peck on something at around 9:00, before going to bed. Do we need to eat at all these times? No. What is true is that, just like Pavlov's dogs, by creating such a routine we have got our body used to being hungry at these times. So, it's as if at 7:00, at 10:00, at 1:00... the bell has been rung for us and we start to salivate. We end up eating, without being hungry, because of a conditioned response. At certain times, our body will release hormones and saliva and make us think that it is time for a snack, for a little bite, for that pastry, for coffee and cake, for hot chocolate. So, just like that, we are Pavlov's dogs, an industry experiment.

As I write this, I am reminded of some moments in my childhood which inspired a tantrum, but for which I am thankful today. In those days, it was normal to eat three times a day, just as our grandparents did (breakfast, lunch and dinner). If, for some reason, I did not have lunch and later asked for food, one of the adults would say to me: "No, young man! You wait until dinner; you can't eat when you're not supposed to". Or maybe the opposite would happen. Perhaps I had "pecked" on something before dinner and when it was time to eat I would say that I was full. I'd then once again hear the adult voices telling me: "See? That's what happens when you stuff your face when you're not supposed to". It's shocking to see how quickly the body adapts to those bad habits and forgets the lessons of our grandparents.

The good old days! We would eat three times. Until the trend for doing it five or six times a day arrived, because otherwise "the body is left without energy and eats the muscle". No more with this nonsense! If that were true, then you and I would die every night. Or what would happen to those teenage sleepyheads who tend to sleep for 12 hours if they're allowed to? Do they die because they don't eat during that time? Should we wake them up every three hours so that they can have a "snack"? It doesn't make sense. We are not bears in hibernation, we don't need to eat so much and so poorly.

I explained it in the previous chapter. When we eat, we put our insulin to work. If we eat more often, well it will have to redouble its efforts. Its production will skyrocket, and we already know the consequences: we will store fat —that's what the excess of glucose turns into— and over time we might develop type 2 diabetes as a result of insulin resistance; our metabolism will be a mess and, as we have created a conditioned response, we will always be hungry. And we will surely crave a nice piece of cake and a cola drink. Sugar! That beauty which stimulates our brain *eight times more* than cocaine. Congratulations.

It has been proven that up to 80 % of the food products found in a regular supermarket contain sugar or some kind of sweetener. Have you checked the pasta sauces which are supposedly savory? There you'll see it. And that is just one example. On my Instagram account (@drcarlosjaramillo) you can find more; there, I tend to publish some posts about jars, cans and packets which are more than suspect: many of them contain tons of the "white lady", even though we believe them to be healthy. Some people say I'm exaggerating. I don't think so. If we were constantly getting healthier and illnesses around the world were decreasing, then it wouldn't make much sense for me to write these lines. But as that's not the case, I suggest we continue.

The food industry is well aware of this: sugar is addictive so they add it to anything they can. It will encourage people to keep eating. So the world is creating an army of food addicts; hunger zombies, the latest creation of our century; they wander like dimwits along the aisles of supermarkets, looking for something to devour. But it's not their fault. It's the result of the system we have invented and accepted. It's the sugary version of *The Walking Dead*.

Now that I am a father of a small child (who I call my teacher), my concern about the way we feed our babies has grown even more. When we are born we need to eat every three hours, we need our mother's milk. But if a mom, as is common these days, cannot produce milk, we have to give the little one the so-called formula. And guess what substance it contains? Exactly. Sugar. The specialist companies in this sector have tried to copy the composition of maternal milk in the products offered on the market. If the former contains a carbohydrate, well they, too, put one in their formula; they said "We replaced that carbohydrate with ours". It seems logical. Again, it isn't. There is no comparison. Lactose in breast milk is not addictive and when the body "breaks it down", it can use it as energy because it comes from the joining of two sugars: galactose and glucose. The latter will provide the baby's cells with energy. For its part, the sucrose we find in formula milks is a mix of fructose and glucose and it does not behave in the same way inside the child's organism. If the word "sucrose" sounds familiar, it is because it is, as a matter of fact, table sugar.

Today, we have children who, from the first months of their lives, are receiving a sweet and dangerous diet. Every three hours, with their formula, they will consume sugar. And they are going to need more as they grow. From a very young age, our children, used to this rush, will look for an ultra-sweet taste. When it's time for their complementary feeding they will not want to eat, they will just cry out for their sweet baby bottle. They will be sugar addicts. And add to this the big business that has been built around infants: yogurts, compotes, smoothies, the list goes on. All of them contain *that* substance. We have, therefore, babies who are joining the ranks of the hunger zombies. How well we're doing!

It sounds a bit apocalyptic, but it's up to us to ensure that it isn't. We can change this. There is a solution. And that's what we will talk about in the next sections. We close off this chapter

by saying that we must reconcile with ourselves by making better decisions when it comes to feeding ourselves. We also need
to forgive ourselves if we are in that spiral of food addiction and
eating anxiety. Let's not think that we lack the will power to stop
eating; as I've said, when we have caused a metabolic disorder in
our body, when sugar is calling out to us, when we have created a
conditioned response, it's hard to escape the weird and powerful
spirit who shouts: "Food, more food!". How wise our grandparents
were for eating three times a day.

Chapter 5

Chronic inflammation

It's important that we understand the significance of the concept which gives this chapter its title, because all all the illnesses that the human body develops will involve some form of inflammation. Let's first talk about the "acute" type. This is the kind we see all the time, the kind that occurs when we are stung by a bee or receive a big blow. The affected area begins to turn red, increases in size, fills with liquid, feels hot, and hurts. Those are the classic symptoms. If, this morning, you banged your shin on the foot of the bed, then you know what I'm talking about. These inflammations are like a big wave which reach their crest and then start to recede until they fade completely. Like the bruise on your shin. To calm the effects caused by these inflammations, we have readily available anti-inflammatories, such as ibuprofen and diclofenac, among many others. Relax, it hurts, but it will be ok.

Chronic inflammation is different. In fact, it is the breeding ground for all the chronic illnesses we are currently suffering from. If its cousin is the big, wild wave which eventually calms and disappears, this is like a constant tide which, after bashing against the wooden dock for so long, eventually breaks it. Chronic inflammation remains over time and is produced by various causes which have affected us for years.

From the moment we are kids we make up part of the modern dietary model which affects our metabolism. We are exposed to a heap of radiation and various chemicals contained in cosmetics, the clothing we wear, soaps, detergents, perfumes. The list is endless. Chronic infections inflame us. We become inflamed due to our poor mentality, not accepting our conscious being, blaming ourselves for everything and thinking that we are simply like this and there is no way of changing. It has been shown that even depressive disorders are related to inflammatory patterns in the body.

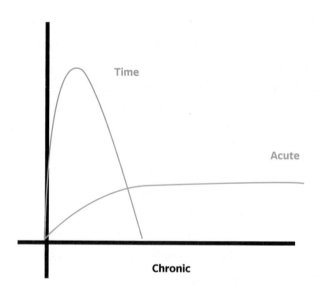

We doctors tend to frequently omit and cancel chronic infections because we don't understand their true clinical reach. Let me talk about one of them, which is very common: oral herpes, better known as "cold sores".

When a person is very stressed, their defenses generally lower and the "cold sore" appears. This is a sign that something in the patient's body is not right. Herpes is a virus which just sits there, hiding, keeping quiet in our organism, waiting for its chance to act. And it almost always comes out to party when faced with stressful situations. Just like oral herpes, there are lots of other chronic infections which we need to be aware of and which appear as a result of the presence of multiple viruses, but there are also chronic fungal infections, such as thrush, intestinal parasite infections, and unidentified chronic bacterial infections.

Chronic infections lead to chronic inflammations, just as allergies do. One of the most well-known is rhinitis (or hay fever), which we see a lot in children and our kids. Aunt Bertha will no doubt tell us: "My dear boy, there is no cure, everyone in our family has it. It's hereditary!" But it's not, auntie. The truth is that hay fever occurs as a result of a constantly inflamed mucous membrane. It is a permanent, constant inflammation, which will generate long-term problems and which is simply the proof that there is a greater process going on inside the body which we are not yet able to see.

Likewise, we have to keep an eye on our gut flora, changes in which are seen ever more frequently in the 21st century, due to two main reasons: an excess of Cesarean births and the exaggerated use of antibiotics. **If the gut flora are in a changed state, this will contribute to bodily inflammation because they will act like a chronic infection. And it will present all the secondary metabolic and biochemical alterations due to its imbalance. The organism will be fighting all day against an inflamed intestine.**

Here's something interesting: a few years ago, many of my colleagues would give off a derisory smirk when I spoke to them about "that microbiome" or "the so-called gut flora". They laughed because they underestimated its importance. Well, today it is a headliner at medical congresses on any specialty. Ah, so it turns out it was important.

As are the so-called "food intolerances", which are different to allergies, and are more visible each day. Although the former do not provoke direct, immediate effects like the latter, they can produce chronic symptoms which can show up to 72 hours after exposure to the foodstuff. If these are present all the time they will be the cause for prolonged, chronic inflammation. I know the effect very well, as I am intolerant to almonds. Yes, those little things I tend to recommend so much. What happens to me is that, between 24 and 48 hours after eating them, I trigger an inflammatory response which causes a slight, but constant, itch in my beard, as well as water retention. I have also had patients who suffer more significant intolerances: some become depressed after eating an orange —it's not a bad joke; it's true— and others suffer panic attacks and hallucinations as a result of gluten. The intolerances I am talking about, could have many consequences.

I also know of another *very* close case. My wife Adriana has suffered an intolerance to eggs which produces eczema on her neck for more than 15 years. After carrying out the necessary tests we found out that gluten —which we will talk about later— and eggs were causing her these symptoms. I had to remove both elements from her diet and correct some secondary intestinal problems caused by the gluten, and her eczema disappeared. Magic? No, we found the leak and fixed it.

The most common way we cause inflammation in our body is through our poor dietary choices. One of those is the continued consumption of vegetable oils rich in omega 6, like almost all those you might have in your house, sunflower oil, corn oil, canola

—yes, don't be shocked—, soybean oil and margarine. Although their packaging states that they are endorsed by the country's medical associations, I'd like to remind you that the industry's companies pay these institutions all over the world. The American Heart Association (AHA), for example, is funded by the corn and canola industry. Terrified?

You'll no doubt be wondering: So omega 6 is bad? No, by no means, it is a fatty acid which is very common in our food, much like its relative omega 3, but the oils I just mentioned are *bad sources* of omega 6. And in excess, it is not beneficial to our metabolism.

As we have mentioned it, let me introduce you to arachidonic acid —an omega 6. Each time we take an anti-inflammatory, we are blocking the so-called "arachidonic acid cascade"—. That is to say that this fellow contributes to the inflammation of the organism and its production will be stimulated every time you consume oils with bad omega 6, like those already mentioned, in excess. In other words, these products should come with a coupon attached to the bottles for a discount on ibuprofen, so that you can take it after using them to cook.

Ideally, we would all have the same proportion of the two omegas, 6 and 3, in our bodies. If you have four times more of the former than the latter, a problem begins to arise. And if we analyze the case of the Western world, where almost all inhabitants have 25 times more omega 6 than 3, well, we are faced with a rather discouraging panorama. The loss of the balance between one and the other is a decisive factor in chronic inflammation and increased cardiovascular risk, and it has an influence on numerous illnesses, such as allergies, arthritis, arthrosis, lupus, cancer and psoriasis, among others. And all of this is produced alongside, as a trigger for or as a result of changes to our hormones, insulin, leptin and cortisol; and an increase in uric acid. Metabolic disaster. We don't know whether the chicken or the egg came first.

We've all heard about the importance of antioxidants. We are told that they are excellent for the body, that they have a number of properties, but nobody understands what they are and what they are for. There are numerous antioxidants: omega 3, vitamins C, E and D —this last one is key to our health—, glutathione and the superoxide dismutase enzyme. And yes, they could well end up being beneficial for our organism. Let's say that the antioxidants are good guys, like the Justice League's Super Friends; and their opposites are the free radicals, who live on the fringes of the law, but it's not their fault. Chronic infections, smoking, radiation, our poor lifestyle and the chemicals we are exposed to all day help to generate lots of free radicals. And when we have more of them and fewer antioxidants, this leads to so-called "oxidative stress", which is a factor in the causes and continuation of chronic inflammation, and in the development of various diseases, especially those which we prefer not to talk about, like autoimmune diseases and cancer.

Have you heard of a telomere? I think perhaps I'm bombarding you with technical terms in this chapter, but let me explain. A telomere is simply one of the ends of a chromosome (you will recall that this is the part of the cell which contains genetic information). It's like the plastic casing at the end of the shoelaces on the shoes you are wearing. Telomeres determine our genetic age, which is different to that which appears on our driver's license or passport. If the free radicals —the bad boys who live on the fringes of the law— are let loose in our organism, and on top of their presence we add a lack of antioxidants in our body and the absence of wise decisions, like a good diet, exercise and meditation, they will drastically shorten the telomeres. And that, of course, will also shorten your lifespan. Perhaps nobody has told you this, but human beings are designed to live for 125 years. They have even done tests on identical twin siblings in which they compare their state of health and measure the length of their telomeres.

The tests show how, in two people with the same genetic code, there can be different reductions in the extremities of their chromosomes. This confirms the importance of the environment in which we live and the choices we make on the modification of our genes. If you have a good memory, you will remember that this is precisely what epigenetics, which we mentioned a few pages ago, studies.

Let the cell die

Researchers have told us that cholesterol clogs the arteries and that produces cardiovascular diseases. True. But that is the consequence. Where is the cause? Upon examining the matter in more detail, we see that, if a patient has suffered from chronic inflammation —the tide which over time breaks the pier— this could cause an ulcer in the artery, and in this little "hole", the cholesterol will attach itself and thus stop the blood flowing. So yes, cholesterol does obstruct the blood flow, but why? Because there was damage to the artery —the ulcer—. What caused it? Chronic inflammation. And how did we come to that? By affecting our metabolism. Where did the metabolic disorder begin? In the mouth, in the bad information we gave our body, a disorder which was enhanced by our misguided way of life.

Chronic inflammation is also related to cancer, which has spread all over the world. This disease is produced when a cell, as a result of structural changes and modifications to its DNA, chooses not to die. Let's not forget that all cells must "die" to make way for a new one, so that there is balance in our organism (this is known as cellular apoptosis). If a cell does not follow this natural process, it starts to multiply, to experience an exponential growth which our body has trouble identifying and which the immune system will be unable to control. In many cases, the cell decides not to die —and causes the illness— due to a series of chronic biochemical changes which stem from, of course, chronic inflammation.

Autoimmune diseases, like rheumatoid arthritis, lupus, Sjögren's syndrome, psoriasis, among others, continue to increase across the planet. When we doctors are faced with a patient who suffers from one of them, we tell them that the origin of their affliction is "idiopathic", meaning that we have no idea where it comes from; that's what they taught us at Med school, and the term sounds very intriguing. It's true, it is hard to establish where the damage originated. What we do know is that many of these diseases also come from chronic infections, which generate chronic inflammation, metabolic, biochemical and physiological disorders, which lead to errors in the body and cause said disorders. They could have been avoided. The truth is that, if the doctor searches patiently for the real cause of the illness in each patient, the panorama will start becoming clearer. Once we know what the origin of your sickness is, we can start to work on it.

For all of the reasons I have laid out, we have to pay close attention to chronic inflammations and remember that we must always keep our body's two largest filters in good condition: I'm talking about the intestine, which we bombard each day with a bad diet and into which we input cheap information, and the mind, which we rarely nurture, because we are always looking towards the outside and we forget to bring our gaze back to our interior to make peace with ourselves. Sometimes, when we look at ourselves in detail, we realize that the stress of work is annihilating us, that, despite having money in our account, we are not happy, that we don't have time —or we don't find the time— for our family, our children, our friends, we don't even set aside half an hour to eat and be thankful for this bounty. And so we realize that we are living a very poor lifestyle. Our mind alters some neurohormonal behavior and from that perspective we are helping with the chronic inflammation. We need to look after both filters, the intestinal and the cerebral. And here it goes again: the most loving way to look after ourselves is to give ourselves a good diet.

The good news, as you already know, is that chronic inflammation does not happen overnight and it can be stopped. But, of course, reversing it will take time. We end the first part of the book with her, chronic inflammation. Don't forget her, she is a leading actress in the development, deterioration and perpetuation of the metabolic syndrome we are trying to cure.

So, have a break, go get yourself a nice, big slice of cake made with vegetable oil and filled with vanilla-flavored cream from a packet and wash it down with a dark soft drink, because your body needs "glucose" so that it doesn't eat your muscle... Hey, yes, I'm kidding. **I'd hope that, after reading this chapter, you would respond to a suggestion like this by saying: "Look, doctor, firstly, it's still not time to eat; secondly, you have drilled into my brain the idea of giving good information to my body, and that piece of cake with a soft drink is not that. Why would I stimulate my insulin and activate my metabolism with such poor information? I appreciate it, but no, thanks".** You are totally right! Would you like to know what you could eat to replace that cheap option of cake and cola? Then keep reading *The metabolic miracle.*

Part two

The metabolic myths

Chapter 6

Foodstuffs

Proteins

For decades, carbohydrates were the kings of the dietary model imposed on us by the false prophets who assured us that fats were the cause of the world's cardiovascular diseases and obesity problems. Remember Doctor Keys' *Seven Countries Study,* presented in the late 1950s; remember the *Dietary Goals for the United States* of 1977, and finally the 1992 food pyramid, invented by the Department of Agriculture in the country then governed by George H. W. Bush.

Backed up, of course, by the caloric evidence —one gram of carbohydrates only contains four calories—, the guardians of health shouted to the world: "Give up fats!". Welcome to the kingdom of cereals, pastas, bread and the rest. However, over time, specialists, nutritionists and people themselves, upon noticing their abdominal roundness, started to realize that these *carbs* were making them fat. That's why they started to turn their gaze to that other macronutrient that wasn't spoken about as much: proteins.

That's how protein-based diets were born. And yes, when people controlled the amount of carbohydrates they consumed and increased their protein intake, their weight began to drop. It was a *boom*. A huge shake-up. Humanity embraced proteins —just as it had previously praised carbohydrates— and there was a surge in eating regimes based on a high intake of proteins. Suddenly, millions of people, especially gym and fitness junkies, were eating meat everywhere, and at all hours.

People were losing weight. Without a doubt. And another erroneous premise took on great importance when interpreted. It was said that protein did not have a glycemic index (GI). Don't forget that this refers to the available capacity of glucose that a person has in their blood after having consumed a foodstuff. Depending on what they ingested, this will be higher or lower. They will have more glucose if they have eaten a slice of cake and less if they chose a serving of broccoli. Therefore, it is totally logical that after eating a nice piece of meat you won't have any sugar in your blood stream. Meat is a protein and is part water, part fiber and part fat. It doesn't contain any glucose! So it is obvious that it doesn't have a glycemic index. But that does not mean it is not going to stimulate the insulin.

Therefore, proteins are declared to be our savior. Not just for their non-existent GI, but also for their thermic effect; in other words, because they raise the organism's temperature. It is believed that if the body generates more heat it will burn a greater number of calories, such that those who follow a high protein diet will rapidly lose weight. It sounds logical, but it isn't true. And, in case it wasn't clear from what I said in the first part of this book, let me repeat: calorie counting does not work.

I suggest we pause once more. Let me ask you a question: Do you remember, in order, which macronutrients increase insulin levels the most? Breathe. Close your eyes. Yes, first it's carbohydrates. Then, *proteins*. Finally, and very minimally, fats. Let's resume. If proteins don't have a glycemic index, using what mechanism can they activate insulin? Using one which starts in your mouth. The excessive consumption of proteins will produce more glucose in the organism.

Many fitness and sports fans fell into the trap of believing that they have to eat a serving of protein every three hours. That's why we see them gnawing on a piece of chicken or snacking on a slice of ham while queueing up at the bank. They believe that if they reach astronomic levels of protein consumption, they will burn more calories and increase their muscle mass. They will manage it to begin with, but it is an unsustainable model. Human beings were not created to eat this way. There is no logic to a person eating five or six times a day, firstly because today food isn't as available, and secondly because it is not natural for us to just eat meat, tuna, chicken or ham; that is a nonsensical diet.

Proteins are necessary for the organism, that is undeniable. Their structure is made up of little bricks called amino acids. Some of these can be produced by the body itself, but many others cannot; that's why it is necessary to eat them. These are the so-called "essential amino acids" (there are also "essential fatty acids", which we have spoken about; omega 3 is one of them). Proteins are necessary. What is unnecessary is eating them excessively. An avalanche of protein brings with it consequences.

Our organism, in the absence of carbohydrates, can create glucose using different sources, like proteins and fats. This process is called gluconeogenesis. If you overdo it with the proteins —by eating chunks of meat every three hours—, this excess will convert into "sugar". But, you will be wondering: What is an exaggerated consumption of protein? It's eating more than 0.8 to 1 gram of effective protein per kilo of body weight, if you don't do any physical activity. Or if you are doing intensive physical activity and you want to gain muscle mass while training, that amount will be more than 1.5 grams of effective protein per kilo of body weight. Note that I am talking about "effective protein" —a term which I will use repeatedly in the following paragraphs—. Let me give you an example: you ordered that T-bone steak you like so much and ate 100 grams. Animal meat has, on average, 25 % effective protein (remember that it is also made up of water, fiber and fat); so you ate 25 grams of it.

How can you calculate, without going mad, how many grams of protein you should consume per day? Follow the instructions I suggested above, or look at another example. Let's suppose that you weigh 80 kilos and you regularly exercise. Ideally, you should consume, more or less, 80 grams of protein a day. So, if you ate 150 grams of steak (37.5 grams of effective protein), 150 grams of chicken (another 37.5 grams) and an egg (which contains 7 grams of effective protein), you will have eaten 82 grams of effective protein. That's fine. "But doctor, you said that it should be 80 grams!". Relax, it doesn't require that level of accuracy, a little more or a little less doesn't make a difference. Don't get worked up. You don't need to take your calculator to the dining table. But that's the suggested balance for someone who weighs 80 kilos and does a moderate amount of exercise. Ok? How much do you weigh? How much exercise do you do? What protein have you eaten today? Do your sums —again, without becoming obsessed—.

Thanks, little rats

In 2005, doctor and biochemist T. Colin Campbell and his son, the doctor Thomas M. Campbell, published *The China study*, a book which became a bestseller, which caught my attention and has acted as inspiration and helped me understand the behavior of proteins. The text examines the relationship between food, diabetes, cardiovascular diseases, cancer and the half-truths which big industry and the scientists they pay tell us. I recommend it.

Throughout its pages, the reader becomes aware of the drama experienced by the former Chinese prime minister, Zhou Enlai, when he was diagnosed with prostate cancer in 1973. He ordered a national study to find out how far this disease had spread in his country and what forms were most affecting its population. China is an ideal nation in which to carry out such tests, because there has been little interethnic mixing, the majority of its inhabitants descend from the Han. This observational study revealed that those groups with the highest cancer rates were those which consumed the most protein. The topic was of great interest to T. Colin Campbell, who focused on testing the possible causes of this finding.

The doctor carried out an experiment with rats to corroborate if proteins could have a direct connection to cancer. He used a very well-known toxin, aflatoxin —which is even found in peanuts— to induce hepatocellular carcinoma (liver cancer) in some rodents. He divided them into two groups. To the first group he administered a certain quantity of aflatoxin and fed them a diet which included just 5 % protein. To the second group, he gave the same dose of aflatoxin, but with a diet of 20 % or more protein. All the rodents in this second group developed cancer, while none of the rats in the first groups showed signs of the illness. The evidence was overwhelming, but Campbell continued with his studies. He then took a group of the rodents affected by the induced hepatocellular carcinoma, maintained the dosage of aflatoxin, but reduced their proteins to less than 10 %. What happened? All of the rats started to show a reduction in the size of their cancer. The tests carried out by the doctor were impossible to question.

However, his findings turned out to be a nuisance to many industries and even to Cornell University, which pulled its funding for a while.

The China study gives us a clear lesson in the importance of protein in our diet, but in the right quantities. An excess of protein will become glucose. If the body does not use it, then it will store it in the form of fat and thus take a sure step on the road to metabolic disorder. I think that much is clear. But Campbell's investigation is also connected to epigenetics, which I talked about at the start of this book. This field shows us how the way we eat, the amount of exercise we do, the exposure to chemicals and medication, the way we relate to others and a number of other environmental factors can have a bearing on the way in which our genes, which we inherit from our parents, can "switch on" or "switch off" when faced with a certain stimulus. So, one of the main epigenetic factors which influences the growth of a cancer, independent of the toxin to which we are exposed, is the amount of protein we consume. **Careful now: I am not stating that protein is a carcinogen. No. I am saying that, if you eat them all the live long day, even while you are reading this book, that excess, coupled with a poor lifestyle —not enough sleep, lots of stress, sedentarism, low self-esteem and little "nourishment" for the mind and spirit— can provoke the stimulation of a cancer.**

As I wrote the last line of the previous paragraph I remembered that one of the other reasons I am writing this book is to try to battle against misinformation. Just like the large media outlets today fight against so-called *fake news*, we should all fight against fake diets, those which put people's lives in danger. One of these is the notorious "carnivore diet", which various bloggers and influencers promote on the internet. They not only claim that humans should only eat animal meat all day, they also dare to say that vegetables are harmful. It is true that there is some evidence to back up the fact that this dietary regime improves symptoms in patients with autoimmunity, but, on the flip side, eating just animal meat increases, in many people, the insulin-like growth factor (IGF-1) and the mTOR pathway, which are pathways which should not be activated due to their high carcinogenic risk. Under no circumstances should you follow this diet, or follow it if you want to tread your path towards cancer. The responsible consumption of meat, in terms of frequency and dosage, alongside following of the recommendations I set out in this book, can be very healthy. Be careful with these fake, risky and illogical diets!

Let's get back to the main point. The overabundance of protein in the diet frequently causes kidney failure, especially with the high doses recommended for the attainment of an increase in muscle mass, which in some cases is as high as three grams per kilo of body weight. The kidneys are like little sieves. Each time blood passes through them, they carry out a "filtration" operation. If a person has exceeded the recommended consumption of protein, the protein will destroy these fine meshes, break them and cause an inevitable kidney calamity. This is a complaint that we doctors tend to worry about plenty, but it isn't the one we most attend to; the problems we see most as a result of an exaggerated intake of proteins are the ones I mentioned in the previous paragraph.

It's best to keep your composure when faced with dietary regimes based on a dominance of the macronutrient we are dealing with here. Do you remember the all-too-famous Atkins diet from the 1980s? It was high in fats and proteins. Did people on it lose weight? To begin with, yes, but 20 days or a month later people stopped losing weight, were riddled with constipation and had the breath of a dragon with cavities. That's where their super-protein journey ended. Over the years, Atkins underwent modifications and became a ketogenic diet, which we will talk about in the section dedicated to fats.

However, throughout the world, there are millions of people totally devoted to their protein-based diet. With this, came a raft of new creations from the industry: zero-calorie protein bars and powders to make "shakes" bursting with the fitness universe's favorite macronutrient. What do these little bars really contain? How can they be sweet and taste of chocolate if they don't contain sugar or cocoa? "But doctor, they taste of chocolate!", you may want to scream, fan that you are of these chewy little bars. Well yes, but what you are in fact eating is a "thing" full of chemicals. Between 75 and 80 % of that sweet treat is made up of them: chemicals!

And it's the same with the magical pixie dust that comes in the magical tub so that you can make magical restorative shakes. That mixture is made using whey —very trendy these days—, which is curdled milk protein. As a macronutrient it has its benefits, there is no denying that. It has a high nutritional value and good bioavailability. However, that shake which tastes and smells of Tahiti vanilla is made up, basically, of chemicals, just like the little bar.

Let's continue with whey. It is one of the proteins found in milk, which also contains others, like casein and lactoglobulins. I said that whey can have its benefits, but it also has its cons. In fact, it's one of the proteins which raises insulin levels the most. That's why, if you excessively consume these powders, using them six or seven times a day, as recommended by your personal trainer or your pal Pete The Muscles, you will be over-stimulating your insulin, which is a hormone which activates every time you eat. You will cause your body to form new forms of glucose, through gluconeogenesis —we mentioned this not too long ago—, as a result of consuming so much protein. So I recommend that you think very carefully before drinking that Tahiti vanilla shake so many times a day.

Plants or animals?

This is a frequently asked question. Is protein from beef better than protein which comes from vegetables? They are both good. As I said before, I'm not going to get into whether being a radical vegan is better or worse than being a self-confessed omnivore. That isn't the discussion being opened up by *The metabolic miracle*. This book needs to be inclusive. But I am going to tell you what I think, what I know and what I understand on the topic. By the way, for many years I have been vegetarian, I don't eat meat because I simply stopped liking it; not because it is a "carcinogen", as many studies at the time claimed. I feel good like this. It was a choice I made after being a meat-eater all my life.

There is a protein which I value highly, and that is eggs, a food which is also a good source of healthy fats and which was given a bad rap for many years. We were all told that it was guilty of causing high cholesterol and other atrocities. Regarding eggs, and about how many we can eat a day —if you aren't allergic to them—, I will speak more at the end of this book. So just take note: eggs are a fantastic source of protein. Add them to your diet.

On the vegetable side of the protein universe we have the legumes: beans, chickpeas, lentils, broccoli, whole oats and mushrooms, for example. Good proteins. And there is another source, much used by vegans and vegetarians, which was even given seemingly miraculous properties for many decades, the soybean. If we examine it in detail, it is clear that it is an appropriate source of protein. "So, doctor, why do you talk about it with an air of suspicion?". Because soybeans and corn are the foodstuffs which have the most genetic variations on the planet. They make up part of the notorious GMOs, genetically modified organisms, or "transgenics". Laboratories and big industry transformed their molecular structure so that their seeds would be more resistant to pests, the weather and other factors which could affect their growth. Soy is one of the molecules which has undergone the most genetic modifications, and the foods or organisms with such drastic variations are closely linked to the development of cancer and many other diseases. I'm not saying that you should forget about soy. I am suggesting that, to avoid problems, if you like this legume so much, then buy it from someone who can certify that it is organic and not the mutant seed which abounds in the market. Certified soy. That way, it will provide a good protein contribution to your body.

Now let's head over to the animal protein terrain. If you are a vegan or vegetarian and you don't eat meat due to your beliefs and because you are against sacrificing animals, I respect your position. I think it is very valid, but here we are covering the whole protein universe; I want this book to be useful for everyone, whatever their dietary, religious or lifestyle choices are.

Let's begin with the "fearsome" red meat. Over the years we have been convinced that we shouldn't eat it because it causes cancer. War was waged on it based on many studies which were full of "evidence". The media published various articles on the issue, but when the investigations which refuted the "evidence" came out and those who had fought against red meat retracted their findings, there was no such media fanfare. Yes, they retracted their findings. You didn't know that? That's the problem: almost nobody knew.

Red meat, beef in itself, is not bad. But it is important to know what we are eating. Livestock in industrialized countries tends to be fed with grains, and a large chunk of these are "transgenic", their molecular structure has been modified by man. They are mutant grains which feed the cows which then become the steaks you will eat. I repeat, this tends to happen, mainly, in the countries from what was previously referred to as the First World: Europe or the United States. In Latin America, livestock is generally fed on grass, which is why the meat consumed in this part of the planet is generally of good quality. And just take a look at the contradictions of our globalized world: **while people in the industrialized nations pay more for meat and dairy products from grass-fed livestock, in Latin America, for some unknown reason, people pay up to three times as much for a piece of Angus-certified meat from the United States, which was most probably fed using genetically modified grain. What are we playing at? The world's gone topsy-turvy.** So what meat should you choose? Grass-fed livestock, the meat we produce in Latin America. Red meat contributes a good amount of protein, as well as beta-Carotene, zeaxanthin, selenium, zinc, lutein, magnesium and iron, and it is less toxic than chicken or fish. How much can you eat? I told you a few pages ago.

The meats which do have a close link to cancer are processed meats, like low-quality or industrial cold cuts, due to the high content of nitrite and other chemicals. But here we also need to make a distinction: an Iberian ham, which has been cured and dehydrated in a dark room and which has matured over a long period of time (12 or 24 months) is not the same thing as those supermarket hams made using "liquefied pork", dyed pinks, full of chemicals and gelatin, with heaps of sodium, and packed in plastic packaging which says: "Fat-free". If you like real ham, if you want to eat good products, if you want to give your body good information, pick the former. If you like poison, buy the latter. And be careful with chorizos or sausages: the majority of those found in stores contain a bunch of "extras" which are not good for your organism. Read the ingredients carefully. Ah, ok, do you want some more surprises? I'm sure you like to accompany your eggs in the morning with a nice side of bacon. Have you checked the ingredients? Well it contains huge quantities of sugar. Don't believe me? Tomorrow, when you go to the supermarket, read the information on the packaging, or check on Google. There you have your bacon.

Another commonly-consumed meat around the world is chicken, which, in the right conditions, is a beneficial protein. Although it's the same as with beef livestock, it all depends on how these birds were raised. If they were fed on grain (transgenic mutants) and grew up in horribly overcrowded conditions, they will not be the best food source for our organism. Ideally, you should buy organic, farm-bred chicken, which wasn't raised in small, prison cubicles, and which ate a heap of vegetables. But the quality of chicken does not just depend on its breeding. Generally, poultry is injected with large amounts of sodium so that it can be transported and frozen without too much fuss. You will end up consuming this sodium when you eat your chicken stew for lunch. How much sodium was it? No idea. There's no way to know. That's why I said that, in terms of toxicity, beef, or other less-consumed meats, such as venison, duck, lamb or turkey, will always be a better choice.

Many people claim that eating chicken is harmful due to the amount of hormones they are pumped with. However, this is a common practice in industrialized countries and not very common in the Latin American market. Carrying out these hormonal treatments costs too much money; which is why it is not the norm in our region. Therefore, if someone talks to you about the "danger of hormones" in chickens, tell them that, at least in our Spanish-speaking nations, the real danger is in the grain used to fatten up these birds.

There is a growing worry around the administering of arsenic in chickens to help with their rapid growth; however, I am unaware of the statistics on the topic in Latin America. Remember that arsenic is highly carcinogenic! "So doctor, can I eat chicken then?". If you are not vegan, and you choose the kind I recommended (organic chicken preferably, or from a known farm), of course, in the correct amounts.

There are other, much-fancied, "clean" —low toxicity— meats, which are appropriate sources of protein for our diet, such as duck and lamb. On the other side of the coin we have pork. Its meat is a great conundrum. While it may have fats which could be beneficial, the problem with pigs is also their diet. The majority of them eat grains. Furthermore, pork is rich in histamine, a molecule which is also present in the human body and carries out many functions; in fact, it operates as a hormone or a neurotransmitter. Histamine is directly related to our body's allergic processes. That's why "anti-histamines" are prescribed for allergic reactions. If pork contains high levels of histamine and you suffer certain types of allergies, it's best not to include it in your diet. And, in general, of all the mass-consumed animal meats, the one with the fewest positives is this one.

I have assisted patients who have told me with a big smile on their face that they have taken a transcendental step in their lives. That they have stopped eating beef forever and are only eating fish because it is "super healthy". Again: in ideal conditions, fish is wonderful, it is an excellent source of protein, and it also has very good minerals, phosphorous and some even contribute omega 3. But what is the current reality of our world? The fish in almost all the oceans and rivers end up feeding themselves on all the trash that we humans have produced in all four corners of the earth. That's why many species are contaminated with high levels of mercury.

In January 2019, I saw a piece in the Spanish economic paper *Cinco Días* which caught my eye. Kiyoshi Kimura, a Japanese millionaire businessman, owner of a sushi chain, paid 2.7 million Euros for a 275 kilogram Bluefin tuna. In the article, the rich businessman said: "I hope that our clients eat the tuna". His intention of pleasing his customers is noble, but it has its risks. When I saw the article I immediately thought that I would include it in the chapter that you are currently reading. The two species which have the highest risk of mercury contamination are swordfish and tuna, large marine specimens. And what about that 275-kilogram fish?! How much of that heavy mineral could it contain?

My recommendation therefore is, if you like fish, limit your consumption of big fish, like tuna; eat it once a month. Salmon is an intermediate species, eat it without going overboard. And if you are one of those who believe that bigger is better, I suggest you set that belief aside and choose the smallest fish species —which are the least contaminated with mercury—. Sardines are a good option, tasty by themselves and rich in omega 3. Small has its charm. Another good option is freshwater fish, as long as you know its origin. Trout, for example, has good protein and a good amount of omegas. Remember that omega from fish is very high quality and provides great benefits to your body. It makes up part of the essential fatty acids.

I mentioned earlier that there are various proteins in dairy products. One of the most important, due to its availability and protein value, is casein. But it's best to keep your eyes open. Casein is like the hot guy from the neighborhood who all the girls want to date, but it turns out that this good-looker is actually a jerk, a cad, a bad egg. What is more important, his Brad Pitt looks or his values and how he behaves? As our parents would tell us: "Weigh it up". Are there more pros or cons? If we're talking about casein, it's the latter. It causes the same damage to our bodies as gluten —wheat protein, which I will talk about later— as both cause what is known as "intestinal permeability".

The intestine works like a juice strainer. Its fine mesh catches the excess of pulp and seed from the fruit and only the juice passes through the sieve. The intestine does the job of filtering: it chooses what the body should absorb and eliminates the rest. Now imagine that the juice strainer, from overuse, starts to break and some larger holes begin to appear in the mesh. Yes, the liquid will still pass through, but it will be joined by residue from the pulp and seeds. The same thing will happen to the intestinal walls when faced with an avalanche of casein: they stop being a good filter, allowing uninvited guests to enter the body, who then cause chronic inflammation and could even trigger immune system responses and lead to diseases such as asthma, acne, insulin resistance and even cancer and autoimmune illnesses, among other diseases. Casein and dairy have an "intimate" relationship with chronic diseases —we will also look at this in detail in a few chapters—. Enough about meat and broccoli for now. Let's get onto the world of fats.

Fats

It all began with a lie, or more precisely, an incorrect interpretation of the evidence. We spoke about it in the opening chapter, in "The epidemic". After Ancel Keys' *Seven countries study* (1958), fat was treated like a murderer, it was blamed for clogging people's arteries and causing cardiovascular problems and millions of deaths. Then the United States Department of Agriculture told the world that it was best to have a diet rich in carbohydrates. That's how the sugar empire began, backed by big industry, strengthened by marketing agencies and held up by the unstoppable global consumption of sugary products. It also kicked off the age of calorie counting. Once again, people pointed the finger at fat: "That fatty macronutrient has a higher calorie content. Don't eat it or you'll get fat! Your cholesterol will increase!", screamed a horde of hysteric nutrition specialists. Again, the industry took advantage of the situation and invented another profitable niche: welcome to the fat-free era.

And what happened in all those years of sugar and low calories? Has the health of the world's population improved? No. You should know that by now, I've already told you. The fat-free, more carbs model brought with it more victims, more cardiovascular problems, more diabetes, more obesity, more eating disorders, more people obsessed with calorie counting and, of course, more companies which pocketed millions of dollars selling their food products for every occasion. The health of those on the planet continues to get worse.

Over these past decades, fat has been a silent witness, a supporting actress, and it has been imprisoned for a crime it did not commit. However, with the passing of time, the dietary puzzle was reshuffled and many studies started to show that, if well used, fats play a valuable part in the diet of human beings. In this chapter, I want to show you why, if we include "good fats" in our meals each day, our health will improve. And, getting back to the question of clogged arteries, remember that, in an unexpected plot twist, the guilty party is actually sugar.

Fats make up part of the lipid group. These, in turn, are divided in two: esters and fatty acids. There are vegetable esters and animal esters; the latter include cholesterol. For their part, fatty acids are divided into saturated, monounsaturated and polyunsaturated fat. I'm sure you've at least heard of the first kind.

I hope you remember something from your chemistry classes at school, especially the renowned "bonds". It's easy, I assure you. Let's begin. Why are they called saturated fats? Because in the carbon (c) chain that makes them up, there is no way of getting any more hydrogen (H) in, there's no space, their structure is, literally, saturated. And notice that there are only single bonds between them. Here's a graphic to help you understand it better.

Saturated

Unsaturated

There are different types of saturated fats. Some are better than others. They are found naturally in dairy or fruit, such as coconuts. And in that oh-so-valuable fluid for the lives of all human beings: breast milk, 27 % of which is made up of saturated fats identical do those in coconuts. I bring up this example in order to start debunking certain erroneous beliefs that Doctor Keys, Aunt Bertha and certain specialists handed down to us as part of their inheritance. One of those is that we should avoid saturated fats because they clog the arteries. If that were true, then perhaps God and nature got it wrong when they put them in the nourishment that a mother gives her child, the first food it receives after coming out of the uterus and into the world. **Given what we have been told for decades, you could say that mothers are criminals for giving that milk with saturated fats in it to their newborns. But wait, that's strange, babies' arteries are not clogged by this milk. Right? Quite the opposite, it gives them the necessary nutrients to grow and begin their lives. And it's recommended by pediatricians, specialists, scientists and all the wise men of nutrition.** Don't forget that. Let's start to bring down these false beliefs.

We have to make an important distinction. The saturated fats you consume in your diet are not the same as those you might have in your blood. Those in your bloodstream are the result of a "maneuver" by the liver in response to a metabolic disorder. Those you eat on a daily basis have anti-inflammatory properties, help to reduce the so-called bad cholesterol and increase the good one, contribute to the creation of various hormones and are vital to the production of a protein which is very important to the pulmonary development of babies during gestation, the pulmonary surfactant. In summary, saturated fats play a favorable role for the body.

Secondly, we have monounsaturated fats. They are called that way because one of the links in the carbon chain which makes up their structure has a double bond (just one). We find them in foods like olives, avocadoes and nuts; and they have multiple anti-inflammatory and immunological benefits. They also help with cardio-cerebrovascular health and the organism's metabolic control.

And the third member of the trio is polyunsaturated fats, which get their name from the fact that their carbon chain includes more than one double bond. This is going to be of interest to you, if only so that you can tell your friends who take a bunch of "omegas". Each carbon in this chain which has a double bond is an "omega". So why is omega 3 called that? Because it is the third carbon on the chain which has the first double bond. The same applies to omega 6, 9 or whichever.

The omega key

As I previously mentioned, omega 3 and 6 are essential fatty acids. This means that the human body cannot produce them, so they must be consumed as part of the diet, as they have beneficial properties. Omega 3 plays an important role as an anti-inflammatory, helps with the creation of hormones and maintenance of cell membrane, but it is also very valuable for cardiovascular protection and brain development. That's why many baby formulas are enriched with omega 3, because it carries out a key role in this last of these processes.

Which foodstuffs contain it? Vegetable sources, such as chia seeds and linseed, or animal sources, such as fish. Where does animal omega 3 come from? Seaweed. Small fish eat seaweed, medium-sized fish eat the small fish, then another bigger one comes along and eats the medium-sized fish and... yes, you've got the picture. In the fish we generally have access to there are two types of omega 3 which we need, EPA (Eicosapentaenoic acid) and DHA (Docosahexaenoic acid), but we could equally consume them directly from seaweed.

Omega 3 has many cousins. One of the most popular is omega 6 —I introduced him to you when we talked about oils—, who, just like Darth Vader, has a dark side. Let's say that good omega 6 comes from primrose and starflower oils, while the bad one is found in canola, soybean, corn and sunflower oils, among others. Within its molecular structure, we find a well-known character, the infamous arachidonic acid, with which our body's cascade of inflammation begins. So let me quickly remind you that a high consumption of omega 6 from the dark side will end up provoking inflammation, which could turn chronic, and the rest of the story you know all too well. By the way, what should the ideal proportion of these two omegas in our body be?

A) 1 to 1

B) 1 to 4

C) 1 to 25

You can check for yourself, but if your answer was "A", I will be very pleased.

We find omega 6 in oils and margarines. The latter were an industry creation, to compete with traditional butter. Margarine is cheaper because it is made from vegetable oils, but in order to get these to solidify, they have to go through a process of hydrogenation. In other words, its biochemical structure is altered. This is how trans fats are formed, which, aside from margarine, are also found in potato chips, cookies, empanadas, frozen pizza, mass-produced baked goods and the majority of supermarket products which we should never ever eat. If there is a terrible fat, it is this one. Please don't consume it. Read the nutritional information on each product carefully.

I know a lot of people are making an effort to follow a healthy diet. My patients tell me: "Doctor, I am healthier than ever, I've changed my habits, now I eat a lot of toasted almonds". Toasted in what?, I ask. "I don't know, I think canola, doc". And canola oil is a bad source of omega 6, so all their good intentions of giving good information to their body with those almonds —which are a great nut for those who are not allergic; I, sadly, am— has gone to pot once it has passed through that process. When an omega 6 from the dark side becomes trans fat, there is no Luke Skywalker to save the person who has consumed it. The body is not capable of eliminating, of metabolically breaking down, the trans fats, and these end up causing a chronic inflammation.

It's likely that you have margarine in your house. You have always used it. And you are probably wary of my words because, what's more, you read on the label that it is healthy and "cholesterol-free". Ok. Let's rewind. If lipids are divided into esters and fatty acids, and margarine is made from fatty acids, tell me where the cholesterol could come from. It's just that the word is linked to fat, which is why you thought: "That's the good stuff!". But no. I like to use this example: it's as if you were to go to an electronics store and find the flat screen TV you want to buy with a notice telling you that it is "cholesterol-free". You'll look for the salesperson and tell them not to try to swindle you, televisions don't contain cholesterol. Well, neither do margarines. They never have.

A new poison?

In the United States in 1948, the well-known *Framingham Heart Study* began, which was carried out in the town of the same name, located near Boston (Massachusetts). The study involved the participation of 5,209 men and women between the ages of 30 and 62, who had never had a cardiovascular problem, stroke or heart attack. This investigation has extended over time, passing through various stages (1971, 1994, 2003), has added other demographic groups and has included the next generations of the first families studied. The conclusions of each stage of the Framingham study have been evaluated and re-evaluated, and in none of the findings over all of these years has there been a single piece of evidence that healthy fats are a cardiovascular risk factor. What would Keys think about all that?

The results of the Women's Health Initiative (WHI) studies, which we mentioned at the beginning of *The metabolic miracle*, and which evaluated a huge number of patients, do not show a risk relation between fats and cardiovascular diseases either. On the contrary, they reveal that the consumption of good fats could be a protective factor for many chronic metabolic disorders.

Another important investigation has been *The Nurses' Health Study*, which began in 1976, is now into its third generation and has involved the participation of more than 275,000 nurses. This study, too, concludes that fats are not a determining factor in cardiovascular diseases.

Renowned doctor, Walter Willett, professor of Epidemiology and Nutrition at Harvard University, has carried out a thorough revision of the medical-scientific literature related to fats and cardiovascular diseases, of clinical studies and the meta-analysis of these investigations, and in no case he has found any evidence that shows that eating fat is bad or that reducing fat consumption has any kind of benefit. In fact, a lot of studies comparing high-carbohydrate, low-fat diets with the opposite, diets high in fat and low in carbs, show that the latter are more cardioprotective, present fewer metabolic complications, and do not provoke diabetes, cerebral thrombosis or heart attacks. It is therefore better to follow a diet which is high in good fats. That's what the evidence says.

Much of the development of the central and peripheral nervous systems is supported by fat molecules. So, if the world continues on this path of fat-free diets, driven by the erroneous belief that fats make us fat, clog our arteries and kill human beings, every day we will see a growth in cases of Parkinson's, Alzheimer's and all the neurodegenerative diseases which have, in fact, increased around the world. Why would we take its essential macronutrient away from our central nervous system? Let it be clear that I am in no way saying that your diet should be based on pork crackling and bacon. Remember that we are talking about "good" fats, like those in avocadoes or eggs, just to name two examples. "But, doctor, fats contain lots of calories! How can they be good?", is something I have heard a lot. Yes, that is entirely true: fats contain nine kilocalories per gram, but so what? Could you please reread the chapter on calories?

Fats are absolutely necessary. And the only way to ensure we have a lot of those that the organism cannot produce is to consume them as part of our diet. **Fats have many benefits: they help to control the metabolism, they contribute to the hormones leading it not being overly stimulated, they have the lowest** effect on insulin levels and, above all, they protect the heart and the brain. **Consume them without fear.** In this book I will explain how. It will do your body good.

On July 18, 2017, the American Heart Association (AHA) brought to light a surprising study in *Circulation* magazine. I say "surprising" because, after reading it, I felt like we had regressed. In this reputable magazine, which belongs to the aforementioned institution, an old discussion is picked up again: in the clogged arteries of those who have suffered cardiovascular accidents and thrombosis there are traces of saturated fats, so the conclusion, to sum up the article's 23 pages, including bibliographic references, is that we should stay away from saturated fats and, amongst those, coconut oil. That text, signed by more than 11 authors, all of course from the AHA, made me uneasy. At the end of the article they recommend a diet low in simple sugars (I couldn't agree more!), low in saturated fats and high in vegetable fats (omega 6) like canola and corn oil (I totally disagree!).

Upon carefully reading the study and checking its sources, it's easy to verify that this "new" evidence is based, principally, on old evidence, three studies which were carried out between 1967 and 1970. That's why I felt we had returned to last century. You might say: "Look, Jaramillo, it was published by the AHA, which is a model the world over, how can you doubt its study? Who do you think you are?". Once again, you are right to be suspicious, but what I am stating is not just nonsense: dozens of doctors around the world expressed their disapproval of this investigation, based on old theories, which ignores, for example, all the other studies I have cited in this section and which show that there is no problem with good fats. They are not responsible for obstructed arteries. The existence of fat in the arteries is the result of a long process, which began with an insulin imbalance, promoted, mainly, by sugar.

What's more, it's strange, but why do they recommend omega 6 oils? If we dig a little deeper, we will discover that some of the nutritionists who work with the AHA are funded by the canola and corn industry, which has lost ground in the global market to other oils, such as coconut oil. But the wide influence and credibility of the AHA means that this speech is spread and that cardiologists and endocrinologists repeat the model and tell their patients to forget saturated fats and consume more canola oil, for the love of God!

To round off the misinformation medley, in August last year, Doctor Karin Michels, associate professor of epidemiology at Harvard, said at a conference at the University of Freiburg (Germany) that coconut oil was "pure poison". The comment had a wide reach, and was published in media outlets such as *The Guardian, The Independent* and *The Washington Post*, and was the main story of the day in many radio stations around the world. Her assertion spread rapidly. Why is it poison? Because, says Michels, it is a rich source of saturated fats. Her media appearances encouraged an interesting debate and raised awareness of this discussion. I, and I say this with no fear, believe in the benefits of coconut oil, I have used it for some time and believe me, I am not suicidal, nor am I trying to poison my wife, Adriana, because I also cook for her using this "horrific" saturated fat. "But Doctor Michels is a Harvard professor!". You're right.

Well let me cite some other Harvard professors. One of them I have already mentioned: Doctor Willett, an epidemiologist and nutritionist who is a leading figure in his field, and who has a very different opinion on saturated fats. Another is Doctor David Ludwig, a great teacher, endocrinologist and author of the successful book, *Always Hungry?* (2016), in which he talks extensively about the benefits of fats. By the way, I love the first sentence of his book: "Most weight loss programs require you to cut back calories. This one won't". I wholeheartedly agree with Ludwig. In conclusion, and getting back to the point, there is nothing to fear about coconut oil or good fats. They are not a poison.

It always strikes me that those who loathe saturated fats tend to crucify coconut oil in their conferences or studies, as if this were the only fat of this kind on the planet. I notice with some unease that some vegan communities and the very same AHA, who are fierce critics of coconut oil, recommend cacao, which is, in principal, another saturated fat. Isn't that a little weird? Well sure, given that cacao can't be used to fry potatoes or to cook, it doesn't represent any kind of threat to the large global superpowers of canola, soybean, corn and sunflower oil. I'm just saying; that's my personal conspiracy theory.

Cholesterol

No doubt several times in your life you have been made to take a test which examines the lipid profile in your blood and measures total cholesterol, which is the sum of the infamous LDL, low-density lipoprotein, the supposed bad cholesterol; VLDL, very low-density lipoprotein, and HDL, high-density lipoprotein, the so-called good cholesterol. What are these three things? Proteins, but *not* cholesterol. What do they do? Transport Mr. Cholesterol, so that total we see in the lipid profile is in fact the amount of cholesterol found immersed in said proteins which transport him. I just wanted to make that clarification.

What's more, as we are told about "good" and "bad" cholesterol, fear is generated and, from that, myths and twisted truths are spread. Cholesterol forms as a result of a metabolic process which happens in our body as a response to something which went wrong or a process which is taking place. And always remember that not you, nor I, nor anybody else eats cholesterol. I shall immediately explain.

Let's check out the transporting trio: LDL, VLDL and HDL. The first, the alleged bad cholesterol, is produced in the liver. It's an important point to clarify, as many people think that LDL is ingested, eaten, that it enters the body in the shape of a greasy empanada, but that is false. This protein is responsible for transporting the cholesterol produced in the liver to the tissues that need it. Why do they need it? To create new cell membranes and hormones, to lower inflammation, for survival.

HDL —or good cholesterol— is the protein which takes the excess, the remaining cholesterol in the tissues, and carries it to the liver so it can "recycle" it or eliminate it in bile, so that the organism can absorb other fats. Because of this removal work, it is called "good", while the "bad" one, LDL, takes the cholesterol to the tissue. But both are "good", they are necessary, they are transporter proteins which help our body.

VLDL —very low-density lipoproteins— are the result of the excessive consumption of carbohydrates and sugars, which end up in the liver. So we therefore need a protein which takes this cholesterol and exports it from the organ to the bloodstream so that it can be stored in tissues in the form of triglycerides, in the subcutaneous fat. I will talk more about these at the end of this section.

Within the HDL (the "good" one), there are some particles which are more efficient than others at removing the excess cholesterol. But don't lose sight of this: when they hand over your lipid profile, they are simply telling you how many particles there are, not how many of the good ones or the less efficient ones you have; they are giving you a consolidated total.

In the composition of the LDL (the supposed "bad" one), there are some big proteins which can store large quantities of fat, which makes them good; and there are other very small ones which can only store a tiny amount. These represent a problem because they are the ones which can stick to the arteries and start to clog them. But when you are given your LDL reading, you can't know what size the particles are.

There is another measurement which, in the majority of countries, including Colombia, is not taken, and that's the RLP, the remnant lipoproteins left floating around the organism, which oxidize and can easily stick together and cause arterial clogging. But the measurement of the very low-density lipoproteins, VLDL —I hope your head is not exploding with all these acronyms and initials, we are nearly done, I promise—, can give us clues about the remnant lipoproteins in your body. If this figure, taking into account conventional lipid profile values, is lower than 20, there is nothing to worry about.

I want to get back to the topic of clogged arteries and the particles I have been mentioning. Firstly, after plenty of studies, today there is sufficient evidence to say that arteries do not get clogged by high or low cholesterol. In fact, 50 % of those who suffer heart attacks tend to have "normal" cholesterol levels. Perfect. So, what was the cause? We spoke about it before: sustained chronic inflammation —produced by metabolic disorders. Remember that said inflammation ends up generating a sort of "ulcer" on the arterial walls, through which the small cholesterol particles filter and then stick, stacking up on the innermost layer of the artery, called the "tunica intima"—. That's how it gets clogged, leading to coronary thrombosis, heart attacks and even death. So it's not a result of cholesterol in the blood; it's the result of having bad particles. We've heard this story time and again: someone goes to the doctor, who tells them that their cholesterol levels are perfect, and congratulates them because the statin —a medication used to regulate cholesterol— is working, but a week later, as they are out enjoying a walk, the person drops dead from a heart attack. How could that happen? I just explained how, didn't I?

"And how am I supposed to know, doctor, what my particles are like? In my country they don't do that sort of test!", you might be crying out desperately. There are solutions, there are other ways to intuit it and analyze it. Keep this in mind:

1 › The first positive indicator is that your HDL (the "supposed good cholesterol") and triglyceride levels have a 1 to 1 ratio. Let me explain: if you have 70 HDL and 70 triglycerides, one could assume that, regardless of the values of your cholesterol, your particles are good.

2 › Another useful clue is to see that the ratio of HDL to total cholesterol is no greater than 1 to 5, otherwise this could be a danger sign.

3 › But you should also keep in mind your insulin levels. If they are good, I congratulate you! You can then assume that your metabolism is under control and that your cholesterol particles are the good kind.

4 › There are other useful indicators that you could ask your doctor to look at, such as the C-reactive protein (CRP) and uric acid.

But please don't forget that all of this needs to be analyzed globally and dynamically, depending on each person's biochemistry. We are all different!

Take a breath. Have a little rest and let's continue with something less technical and more from the world of myths. For years Aunt Bertha has led us to believe (you, me, everyone) that high cholesterol is a family problem, that it is hereditary and there is no way on earth that it can be fixed —on my YouTube channel I have dedicated an episode to this, I suggest you check it out—.

Actually, some doctors also tell their patients that. But it's not like that. Only 5 % of all cases of high cholesterol has a family origin, the other 95 % are due to acquired causes. Without going into too much detail, that hereditary cholesterol tends to be excessively high, more than 500 or 700, and it is hard to control. Some cases are truly dramatic and involve children dying at a young age because they produce so much cholesterol that it is simply impossible for their body to handle.

Acquired causes, which are the most common, are generally due to a poor lifestyle (poor diet, too much sugar, not enough exercise, too much exposure to radiation, lack of personal motivation) and chronic infections, because the lipoproteins have antimicrobial properties. Let's say that you suffer from repeated urinary infections, which is a sign of chronic infection. In order to control them, your body will try to produce more lipoproteins and so your cholesterol will start to rise. What caused it? That damn chronic infection.

Another acquired cause is hormone deficiency. Don't forget that cortisol, estrogen, progesterone and testosterone are produced from cholesterol. If a woman enters her menopause and stops producing her hormones, the body —in a natural response— will say: "No way, we have to create more cholesterol, we can't let her down!". So the woman will produce more LDL, the lipoprotein which takes the cholesterol from the liver and transports it to the tissues so that, in this case, more estradiol or estrogen can be produced. As this mechanism begins to carry out its functions, the woman will have elevated cholesterol levels. And the solution would not be to give her statin; the medication for lowering them. The only solution is to find the causes of this behavior in order to know how to correct it. Find the hole and cover it up!

Before continuing with triglycerides, I want to reiterate that the state of your health is not caused by the absence of some form of medication. Your high cholesterol is not due to a lack of statin.

In fact, no study has been able to prove that this reduces the risk of cardiovascular or cerebrovascular events. The latest investigations prove that, every day, statins cause more harm than the benefits they provide. And that's not to mention their side effects (like muscular pain) and their contribution to insulin resistance. Does that not seem like a contradiction to you? Lots of patients experience elevated cholesterol levels due to insulin resistance; however, their specialists give them a medication which will worsen the case. Well... now they have created a patient (a client) for life.

Triglycerides

Everyone has something to say about them. But not many people understand them. I tend to say that triglycerides are like that slightly weird, estranged uncle, who is a bit of a freak, doesn't go to the family gatherings and who many label as "bad" because they don't really know him. To begin with, and let me make this very clear, triglycerides are not the product of the fats you consume; they are the result of an excess of carbohydrates, especially the fructose and simple sugars you include in your diet.

Carrying on from what I told you before, if your carbohydrate consumption is too high, the very low-density lipoprotein (VLDL) will form in your liver, and it will have the mission of transporting the "fat" which has been formed there to the bloodstream. It exports it in the form of triglycerides. All good so far? These, for example, are what cause the infamous fatty liver, which, as its name suggests, is evidence that too many lipids have accumulated in this organ. This is a condition which has increased the world over and which produces non-alcoholic fatty liver disease. Currently, this is the main cause of cirrhosis, an illness which, decades ago, was solely reserved for alcoholics and unruly spirits. Another warning sign. And how did this all begin? Tie the loose ends yourself, it isn't hard.

Perhaps you like *foie gras*, which is nothing more than the fatty liver of a duck or goose. I suppose you know how it's made. In order for these birds to develop that fatty liver, they are fed on sugary syrups. Did you get that? Sugar! The industry knows that very clearly. Although neither you or I are ducks, if we end up with a fatty liver it will be as a result of the same thing, the excess of sweet foods we are consuming. The strange thing is that, although we know the cause, the main recommendations we doctors give our patients suffering from this disorder is: "Sir, stop eating saturated fats, that is the root of your problem". Or we blame the genes, their inheritance: "Ah, of course, your father suffered from the same thing, there's the reason!". An excess of glucose caused the fatty liver.

Going back to measurements, tests and triglycerides, if these are showing elevated levels, be in no doubt: this is an unmistakable sign that your insulin levels are also high, which means that there is a metabolic disorder inside your organism. Let me test your memory again: What should the ratio of HDL (the so-called good cholesterol) to triglycerides be? Yes, very good, 1 to 1. If the first measurement is 70, the second should be close to that number. A ratio of 1 to 2 is still acceptable, but if your HDL is measuring 50 and your triglycerides 200 (1 to 4), there is a higher risk of a cardiovascular event. This suggests that you have bad HDL and LDL (bad cholesterol) particles, which trigger chronic inflammation, which can in turn clog your arteries. Any measurement of 1 to 3, or more, should warrant your attention.

However, if you go over everything that we have outlined in this chapter, you will understand that LDL, which for many people is the bad guy, the villain, the filthy scumbag of the cholesterol world, is not responsible for the conditions which are killing humanity.

In this book we have spoken about the factors which disrupt the metabolism. Some signs of metabolic syndrome are obesity, high blood pressure or low HDL levels, among others. Metabolic syndrome has an influence on cardiovascular and cerebrovascular diseases. Diabetes, prediabetes, Alzheimer's and many more. But notice that LDL (the "bad guy") alone, looked at in isolation, is not criteria for determining metabolic syndrome or cardiovascular illnesses —which are what cause the most deaths around the world—.

However, this dangerous, moody guy, LDL, is what cardiologists take into account when prescribing medication to lower cholesterol, because it allegedly clogs the arteries. It shouldn't be this way, but behind everything there is a wonderful industry which needs to sell its pills, so it needs to ensure that they are consumed. And how does it promote this consumption? By confirming that cholesterol is the bad egg.

Fats have been suspects forever; they have been blamed, condemned, without an exhaustive revision of the evidence, just as laid down by Professor Willett, but in this century they have a right to appeal and get out of prison. Some steps in that direction have been made. In the United States' new dietary guidelines, published in 2015 and valid until 2020, it is now recommended that fats not be excluded from our diet, and that we should consume a minimum of 35 % fats. That is encouraging news. The strange thing is, that in the midst of this progress, studies like that presented by the American Heart Association (AHA) in 2017 sow the seed of doubt or tell us: "Fats, ok, but make sure they are omega 6 fats from canola and corn oil". Which is a fairly unhealthy invitation, taking into account what I have told you.

I will be satisfied if, at the end of this section, you have understood that: a) fats are not bad; b) they are necessary for your body, although c) there are fats which are beneficial (like coconut, cacao and avocado) and others which are not (like the omega 6-rich oils) and d) eat the correct amount! Everything in excess is bad.

Thanks, Charlie

I want to finish this section by telling you a story that I really like; it's the one about an American boy called Charlie, son of movie producer Jim Abrahams (*Top secret,* 1984). In 1993, when he was a baby of just 11 months, his epileptic fits were uncontrollable. Medication had contributed little to improving them. So, desperate, his parents decided to turn to a dietary regime about which few people knew, called the ketogenic diet (or keto). One month later, the infant's fits had disappeared and he no longer took any medication. In 1994, his parents decided to start the Charlie Foundation for Ketogenic Therapies, to help more children suffering from epilepsy and other diseases —you can find full details of the story in the hundreds of articles online or on the foundation's official website—.

Why am I telling you about Charlie and the ketogenic diet? Because this diet recommends a dietary model based on 70 or 75 % healthy fats, 15 or 20 % proteins and less than 10 % carbohydrates. You might be thinking that this is suicide. No, it's quite the opposite, it's an invitation to a better life. The level of glucose you will receive with this diet is very low. Remember that glucose is your main source of energy and is stored in the liver in the form of glycogen. If your glycogen reserves vanish very quickly, your body must switch on the second "turbine", thus using all of the energy that you have stored in your body and between your organs in the form of... fat! Isn't this mechanism magnificent?

Your organism enters the ideal metabolic phase. It produces energy from fat, through compounds called ketone bodies. That's where the name of this diet comes from. This diet was very popular around the world at the beginning of the 20th century and proved beneficial in cases of epilepsy and obesity, but several decades later, when the medication boom began, anticonvulsants appeared and turned into a multi-million-dollar industry. The benefits of the ketogenic diet were forgotten.

But in the early 1990s, Charlie Abrahams' case came to light and keto made it onto the news and into the newspapers, and medical communities began to take an interest in the topic again. Since then, there are more studies each day on the positive effects of the state of ketosis on the body, and its benefits for the metabolism, controlling insulin, reversing Alzheimer's, Parkinson's, mitochondrial diseases, epilepsy and autism, for mental clarity, for weightlifting, through the natural incitement of the growth hormone, for various types of cancer, for obesity, and lowering blood cholesterol and cholesterol plaques, among many other things.

Right now you will be shouting out in excitement: "Say no more, doctor, I'm going to immediately start training my body to reach ketosis and that's as far as I'm going with this book!". Hold on a minute. The benefits of the ketogenic diet are undeniable. I recommend it. Dozens of celebrities around the world proclaim its advantages, but heed this: it requires a great deal of will power because, with keto, it is all or nothing. It needs to be perfectly balanced, otherwise it will all be wasted effort. It can take between 2 and 15 days for you to enter into "ketosis" after following the diet word for word. But then you pass a bakery which sells that slice of apple pie that you love so much, and you take a bite (one measly bite!). Bye bye ketosis. It's that extreme. So relax, and let's continue with this book, I'll offer you some other, less demanding options. I only tend to recommend this diet —which, I repeat, has many benefits— to my patients with degenerative diseases, some forms of cancer and epilepsy.

In conclusion: don't remove fats from your diet. Don't count their calories, it's not worth it, they contain more than double what carbohydrates contain (9 kilocalories per gram). Not everything is cholesterol's fault. Don't get caught up in the cheap fat-free philosophy. And keep in mind that the measure of consumption and calculation of your fats should be carried out by a suitable professional. Can you consume good fats uncontrollably? No. What good fats should you include in your diet? Here I outline them so that you don't forget.

Fats to include

Olives, olive oil, coconut oil or coconut itself, avocadoes, avocado oil, walnuts, cashews, pistachios, pecans, macadamia nuts, almonds, chia seeds, linseed, sunflower seeds, sesame, eggs, salmon, trout, cacao, pine nuts.

Fats not to include

Peanuts, peanut butter, sunflower, soy, maize or canola oils, margarine, vegetable spreads, trans fats, hydrogenated or partially hydrogenated fats, industrial fried foods.

Carbohydrates

I am going to tell you something that might perplex you. The basis of a human being's diet, with which we can control our metabolism, lose weight, cure ourselves of diabetes and improve our cholesterol levels, are carbohydrates. Now you will be wide-eyed and wondering: "What are you saying, doctor? You've just spent the whole book warning us that they are bad and stimulate insulin! Have you gone mad?". No. I'm talking about the best carbohydrates on the planet, *vegetables*. The problem is that we have got used to thinking that bread, grains, fruit and sugar are the only representatives of this group of macro-nutrients, but, as we have already seen, they have been the cause of the growth of chronic heart, brain and metabolic problems around the world and are the reason you are reading these pages.

Is lettuce a carbohydrate? Yes. Popeye's spinach? Yes. The broccoli that Aunt Bertha loves so much? Obviously. The structure of carbohydrates is made up of a simple union of carbon (c), hydrogen (H) and oxygen (o). See the following graphic.

Linear chain conformation **Haworth projection** **Chair form conformation**

And they are divided into two families: simple and complex. The former includes glucose, fructose or galactose, which are sugars which preserve the structural basis of carbs. Complex carbohydrates, for their part, are made up of a chain of various sugars. That's the simplest explanation and the one which should suffice for us.

Before we continue with this section, I want to reiterate the central idea of its first paragraph: believe me, it doesn't matter if you are a vegetarian, vegan or meat-eater; it doesn't matter what regime you follow, what does matter is that you understand that the greatest riches for a human being's diet come from what the earth provides for us, from those colorful vegetables that grow out of the ground. These will provide the necessary amount of nutrients, because not only do they include carbohydrates, they contain minerals, vitamins, antioxidants and anti-inflammatory properties. Don't forget it. Make these the basis for each meal.

Getting back on track. Carbohydrates are not "bad". But we have taken to consuming them in the wrong way. For example, we eat an excess of complex carbohydrates like starchy products, including potatoes, yucca or plantains. "Are plantains bad, doctor?". No, nor are potatoes or yucca bad, but what is bad is eating them in excess and all day. The same recommendation applies to the consumption of grains such as quinoa, amaranth and rice, among others. "Rice, doctor? But Chinese people also eat them all day and they are skinny". Firstly, Chinese people also have other sources of food and they consume lots of vegetables; secondly, they are skinny because that is their physiognomy; thirdly, they are very active people and rice (which is glucose) behaves very differently to the poison afflicting our planet. However, as you will have read at the beginning of *The metabolic miracle*, today a high percentage of the Chinese population has diabetes (10.9 %, according to the International Diabetes Federation 2017 report), worrying figures considering that forty years ago, before the dangerous carb which I will talk about in the next chapter arrived in the country, only 1 % of the population suffered from it.

You don't have to load your plate up with the carbohydrates I just mentioned; on the contrary, fill it with vegetables of various colors, loaded with nutrients. You don't need to eat them six times a day. The key is to find a balance. You don't have to eat fruit every two hours either, or drink an excess of fruit juices, and less still, alcoholic beverages. Take note: the best thing to do is make good decisions. Carbohydrates in excess raise insulin levels, and if this has to work extra shifts, it will cause all that glucose you are consuming to turn into fat.

Table sugar, honey, cane sugar and lactose are carbohydrates. These, we have been told for decades, are the most appropriate available energy source for the organism. And, on hearing this, all professional sportspeople —cyclists, athletes, triathletes, soccer players— based their diets on this assertion. Many of my patients are, in fact, high performance athletes and, although it sounds hard to believe, they suffer from prediabetes or diabetes. Why? Due to their excessive consumption of carbohydrates, based on a belief that this is the only way their body can have sufficient energy. That's like continuing to put gas in your car when the tank is already full. It happens to sportspeople. It happens to all of us living in the West, including the inhabitants of the Old Continent. We consume too many carbohydrates and, above all, too much of one which is the worst of all, one which you like a lot and which I will finally talk about at the end of this section —yes, I am intentionally building up your expectations—.

What do I recommend? Your base carbohydrates should be vegetables of varying colors —I repeat—, you should carefully control your consumption of bakery products, and, yes, eat one of those starches that you like so much (rice, potatoes, yucca, green plantain) in some of your meals, but not all.

Other very good carbohydrates are the world-famous "fibers", which are found in vegetables and some grains. There are two types of fiber: soluble and insoluble. The former dissolve in water. They are fermented by the colon's bacteria and create a thick, gelatinous substance in the digestive tract. The latter do not dissolve, the vast majority do not ferment in the colon —there are exceptions— and they provide volume and mass to the fecal matter.

Soluble fibers are important because, as part of their fermentation process, they produce short-chain fatty acids. These are vital nourishment and a source of energy for the intestine's cells. They have an anti-inflammatory effect, improve sensitivity to insulin, help lower the possibilities of neurodegenerative conditions and help with the appropriate production of LDL; they are also crucial in managing chronic inflammatory diseases in the colon —the large intestine— such as ulcerative colitis and Crohn's disease—. One of these fatty acids is butyrate, which plays an important part in resistance to stress and the immune response, and contributes to many metabolic functions. Soluble fibers have also proven to have protective benefits against chronic cardiovascular diseases.

For their part, the vast majority of insoluble fibers —apart from resistant starches, which I will immediately go on to talk about— are of low fermentation. These add volume to stool, improve the frequency of said stool and, unlike soluble fibers, do not generate fatty acids.

What are starches? They are large glucose chains, found in plants, which are good for your diet. Amylase, a protein produced by us humans, helps us to "break down" the starches in the organism and make them more easily digestible for the intestine. Resistant starches —which are insoluble fibers with special characteristics— have a distinctive feature, which is that they can be fermented by the gut microbiota (or flora) in the colon to produce fatty acids, like the aforementioned butyrate.

Resistant starches also help with the absorption of numerous minerals, such as calcium, improve intestinal motility (bowel movements) and the balance of gut flora, contribute to resistance and sensitivity to insulin and to the reduction of cortisol in the mornings —which can sometimes produce elevated morning glycaemia levels in people with good eating habits—. What foods are they found in? Green plantain, potatoes, yucca, tapioca, green bananas and some legumes.

Fiber should always be part of your diet, but it should be consumed in moderation —anything in excess is bad; anything—. It is found in the previously mentioned starches, in fruit, in vegetables, especially those with green leaves, in berries, and in seeds and nuts, like almonds, chia or linseed.

There are various ways to divide and differentiate carbohydrates; I like to do it like this, 1) simple: sugars, honeys, syrups and alcohol; 2) complex: wholegrain, cereals, and 3) starches. This classification allows for us all, doctors and patients, to carry out the task of finding the correct balance, depending on what each person is looking for.

And, if you want my opinion on what should be the hierarchy of carbohydrates in your diet, I repeat that top on the list should be non-starchy vegetables, like cruciferous vegetables (broccoli, cabbage, sprouts, cauliflower, radishes, turnips, among others), kale, spinach, tomatoes, lettuce, chard, carrots, radishes —and a very long etcetera—; then fruits and starches (ideally resistant).

Finally, you have to be very careful with your consumption of refined flour, and understand that white and wholegrain bread raise insulin levels in the same way. I know that half of humanity prefers wholegrain bread because they believe it is healthier and they can eat it without limits. That is false. Don't lose sight of the fact that said refined flours —white bread, cakes, pizzas, pastas— have the capability to raise your insulin levels ten times more than sugar.

The same thing happens with fruit. The World Health Organization (WHO) recommends we eat between seven and nine servings of fruit and vegetables, but does not explain how, or which ones. The WHO's intentions are very good: to try to encourage the world population to consume good carbohydrates, but there have been many problems with the interpretation of this recommendation. What to do? My advice is, if you already know you have metabolic disorders, then eat fruit once a day; that's enough. If your metabolism is regulated, you can eat one or two servings. But the ideal thing to do would be to consume seven servings of vegetables a day, that is to say large servings of them in your three daily meals; and one or two of fruit, ideally in the morning, but not in between meals, rather as part of them. Fruit is not bad; what is bad is the habit of eating it all day, at any time and in any quantity. What does cause problems is juice. I will explain. Let's move on to the next section and we will discover together the most dangerous player in our diet. Ready? You might have trouble believing me. Perhaps you won't want to.

Fructose

Here we are. We got here. I introduce you to this book's lethal protagonist. Why, if it's a carbohydrate, did I not include it in the previous section? Because it deserves its own section. Fructose is fruit sugar —it is a monosaccharide—. And we have always been told that it is fantastic, necessary and completely healthy. At the end of the day, apart from Snow White, nobody has claimed any kind of fruit poisoning. But it's time to raise our voices.

Towards the end of the 1930s, before the Second World War, an average person would consume more or less 15 grams of fructose a day. They would take it in directly from fruit, biting it, sucking it, chewing it. After this conflict, which marked the history of humanity, the average consumption of fructose was between 35 and 40 daily grams. Today, in the 21st century, in such a modern, advanced, fat-free, light and "healthy" era, it is estimated that an adolescent could consume between 75 and 80 grams of fructose a day, five times more than 80 years ago. These figures are not a huge revelation. They don't tell us much. But they give us hints about the increase in its ingestion. Let's get down to business.

First let me remind you how our organism absorbs glucose, so that we can then see how fructose operates. How does that sound? It'll be a kind of summary of everything you have read so far. Let's talk about rice (a cereal, a carbohydrate), which you and Chinese people like so much. Let's say that all that rice you ate for lunch provided 100 grams of glucose to your body. Eighty percent of it will be distributed to your organism's cells to supply them with energy. I explained this earlier, cells need this "gasoline". The glucose will provoke the pancreas (a gland) to produce insulin (a hormone) so that it can regulate and administer the glucose. This mechanism sends a signal to the leptin (the hormone which gives the "don't eat any more, you're full" order), which begins to take note of how much food is coming in and sends a message to the brain saying: "Watch it, the food is arriving!".

The other 20 % of those 100 grams of glucose you consumed with your rice makes its way to the liver, where it is stored in the form of glycogen. Remember that this organ can only store a certain amount of glycogen; if its limit is reached, the rest will be exported to the liver in the form of very low-density lipoproteins (VLDL), which will form triglycerides in the tissue, and that's how the fat in your body increases. So that reserve, in the form of lipids, will take shelter in the tissue for use later. All good so far?

Human beings store fat in order to be able to make use of it in the event that we do not have any food available. The body is wise, it's not wasteful, it's thrifty, it's always thinking about saving some of the energy we supply it with when we eat. Take note that this was initially glucose, but that it has now been turned into fat. Ok? This bodily mechanism of resorting to the fat and transforming it into glucose is called gluconeogenesis; "gluco", from glucose; "neo", meaning new, and "genesis", meaning creation.

If there is no food, the body accesses this fat which we have saved, those valuable funds, to produce energy. **That is how the nomads survived —they didn't have supermarkets or home delivery—. They couldn't eat every three hours, like the 21st century's professional athletes, because they didn't have available food sources all the time. They didn't eat energy bars, or Tahiti vanilla-flavored proteins from a tub, or croissants, and they lived! They didn't even know if they would be able to eat the** following day, and they didn't die! Why? Because of what I am trying to explain: they had energy reserves in their bodies in the form of fat in their tissues. Just as you do, and just as I do. That is how glucose storage works.

Now let's examine the other case. What happens with fructose? Have you ever heard of a bad shortcut? If you consume 100 grams of fructose from apple juice, it turns out that 100 % (all!) of it will head straight to the liver. None of it will go to the cells to act as an energy source. Let me make this very clear: fructose *does not* give your body energy. Remember that when glucose arrives at the liver, it does so with prior notice, it knocks on the door and is let in. Ok, if we're getting technical, glucose uses a receptor and a transporter in order to enter the liver's cells. What does fructose do? It enters using passive transport. It silently sneaks in, without warning.

When the liver receives this 100 % of fructose which arrived without warning, it requires a lot of energy to process it. It activates other mechanisms in the body, stimulates the production of uric acid, which causes so much inflammation that it can lead to high blood pressure as it lowers the levels of nitric oxide —discovered by scientist and Medicine Nobel Prize winner Louis Ignarro—, which is vital for the proper functioning of the arteries. Faced with the unexpected visit of this fruit sugar, the liver can do little; however, it stores a small amount of it in glycogen. But the rest —that is to say, almost all the fructose— has to be exported in the form of VLDL and triglycerides to generate fat. Take note, therefore, that glucose and fructose follow a different journey and assimilation path in the organism.

I spoke not too long ago about the huge growth in non-alcoholic fatty liver disease around the world. I told you about fatty liver (and *foie gras*). This is formed, precisely, due to an excess of fructose. With its impetuous arrival, the liver is forced to carry out so-called liponeogenesis; in other words, there is a "new formation of fat". It makes sense. If the body no longer has space, no more available "pigeonholes" in its organic board for storing glucose, the only thing left to do is lipneogenesis. This converts the orphaned glucose into lipids. The remaining amount will be exported as fat in the tissues, but it will also form visceral fat, fat stored within the organs. This generates the unpleasant fatty infiltration of muscle and fatty pancreas, which bring with them risks for your organism and can be decisive in the creation of chronic and cardiovascular diseases.

This is the origin of one of the final complications of type 2 diabetes, known as "beta-cell failure", which occurs when the pancreas, which has filled with fat, cannot produce insulin. The illness is now no longer caused by the excess of this hormone, but rather the opposite. The gland cannot create it. At the end of the day, the result is the same.

There are some unmistakable bodily signals which show if somebody has consumed a lot of this fruit sugar over the years. Let's talk about Uncle Pete, Aunt Bertha's husband, and his belly. The good man has a rather pronounced abdominal circumference, much like Jiggs, star of the comic strip, *Bringing up father*. His experienced belly is strong: if someone touches it they will notice that it doesn't sink in, like a well-inflated ball. It's the typical beer belly, the kind that many men like Uncle Pete say they have cultivated with pride —they should, on the contrary, be worried about *that* thing they have cultivated—. Their belly is the way it is because it contains a large amount of visceral fat. Be sure to tell Uncle Pete that this is the result of an excess of fructose in his diet. Those people, on the other hand, who are chubby, or who have "spare tires" around their abdomen, also owe this to the consumption of carbohydrates, but especially starches and grains (in other words, to the overabundance of glucose in their diet), and not fructose.

Tell it like it is

Perhaps Uncle Pete might defend himself and say that he never consumed enough fruit or juice to have cultivated his visceral fat belly as a result of fructose. "I don't get it, nephew!", he'll say. "Remember, uncle, all that white sugar you added to your coffee, to your 'healthy' infusions and which you ate as part of Aunt Bertha's cakes? Well, there's the result". Yes, table sugar, refined white sugar, that elegant little thing, the renowned sucrose, is half glucose and half fructose. There's your answer, Uncle Pete.

Let me give you an example. If you, like your uncle, consume 100 grams of table sugar, keep in mind that 50 % of it is glucose and the other 50 % is fructose. What route will the glucose take? Eighty percent of it will head to the cells to produce energy; the remaining 20 % will head to the liver, knock on the door, ask permission to come in and will then be converted into glycogen. On the other hand, the remaining half of those 100 grams of sugar, which is fructose, will go directly to the liver, enter unannounced and without knocking on the door, and will make the liver get to work frantically. Do you get what I'm telling you? The fructose is right there, in your table sugar. Half of those three teaspoons that you put in your kid's chocolate milk at breakfast is fructose. Half of the teaspoons you added to your coffee is fructose —by the way, good coffee doesn't need sugar—. Every day we consume fructose, even if we don't eat a single apple.

And, to top things off, 80 % of the products we find in our supermarkets contain added sugar —like the tomato sauce you used yesterday to make your pasta—. It's a rather discouraging panorama, because almost all of the sweeteners we use are half glucose and half fructose. "But, doctor, I use honey from the Hidden Forest!". Honey is glucose and fructose. "But, doctor, I use organic raw sugar cane!". Very good, it's really tasty, but it is glucose and fructose. Almost all the calories in the planet's natural sweeteners are part glucose and part fructose.

One of the worst sweeteners, which has become very popular around the world and which is recommended by nutritionists and some of my counterparts, is agave honey or syrup. Those who sell it assure us that it is "especially for diabetics" because it has a low glycemic index (GI). I know you have a good memory and will remember that this term alludes to the capacity that a glucose molecule has to be available in the blood after you consume it. The terrifying thing is that the composition of agave syrup is 20 % glucose and 80 % fructose. It has more of the latter than refined sugar! So, if someone tells you that agave syrup is "ideal", tell them that it is, "ideal for becoming diabetic". Be careful with those truths which aren't true and which are plentiful in the dietary world.

There's one protagonist we've not yet mentioned and, although it is not as fashionable as agave syrup, it is very popular: high-fructose corn syrup, or HFCS —55 % fructose, 45 % glucose— which, as it is cheaper than cane sugar, is used for everything. Its perception of sweetness is up to ten times higher than that of sucrose. And I repeat, it is cheaper, a quality which counts for a lot with the large food companies who need sweeteners.

I find it unacceptable that, in supermarkets, in the organic, healthy and even "functional" sections, they sell packets of pure fructose powder, claiming that it is the best option for those who suffer from diabetes because, again, it does not have a glycemic index. And on the packaging we can see that they are endorsed by the diabetics and endocrinology associations of numerous countries. The GI thing is true, the index is zero, but that does not mean that this powdered fructose is good for you and that it does not affect your metabolism.

Perhaps, after reading all that, you might want to ask me the following question: "If fructose does not have a glycemic index, how will it stimulate or raise my insulin levels? How can it produce diabetes? It's illogical!". **Look, fructose does not generate an immediate "spike" in insulin levels because it goes directly to the liver; as if it were invisible to the pancreas. And, worse still, the leptin doesn't detect it. Fructose is like a sugar from the** *Mission Impossible* **crew: it filters through, infiltrates and goes undiscovered.** But an excess of fructose will end up affecting your metabolism. Insulin resistance is produced at two moments: through the inflammation generated by the production of uric acid, from the inflammation of certain proteins, such as JNK1, and from the moment at which the exportation of the triglycerides is generated. It's a delayed effect, but one which is maintained easily over time, making it very effective in producing the insulin excess which could possibly lead to resistance.

That is one of the great dangers of fructose: that its presence goes unnoticed. I'm sure this has happened to you: after a nice, bountiful and enjoyable lunch with friends or family, someone on the table orders dessert. Although you've had enough, you feel that there is still space for that tiramisu you love so much. And you eat it. And you enjoy it. And you don't feel full. You could even eat another. It's as if you had a stomach for savory food and a stomach for sweet food. Almost like cows, who have four. This happens because, like I said, fructose is not perceived by the leptin. There is nobody to send the signal to the brain saying: "No more food!". It's as if that dessert never existed. As if you had made a bank transfer but the system never registered the transfer. But your body is paying the price.

By the way, how many juices did you drink at that lunch? Because there's another habit which affects the metabolism, and a lot. We grew up hearing: "Don't drink soft drinks, drink juice!". I'd suggest you don't drink either. "No, doctor! I'm closing this book, this is the last straw, juice is the healthiest thing in existence!", you'll no doubt want to scream. I'm sorry, but no. Juice, at the end of the day, is pure, loose fructose. When you blend the fruit and pass it through a strainer and throw away its pulp, the only thing left in the glass is a liquid containing vitamins, minerals, a nice taste, water and loose fructose. I think you are already pretty clear as to its journey through your organism. Take note of the fact that the pulp of the fruit will help with your glucose intake and the benefits it brings to your gastrointestinal tract. But the pulp was left in the strainer. And even if you don't strain the juice, this fructose is going to be loose, separate from the pulp.

The two juices which cause the most problems are, of course, everybody's favorites. Orange juice, which tends to be the perfect breakfast partner for tens of millions of people around the world, and mandarin juice, the one which many people order at restaurants because they have quit soft drinks and are starting a healthier, lighter life —and which is really expensive—. Before you well and truly abandon your reading of *The metabolic miracle*, I'm sure this news is very troublesome for you, that you perhaps squeezed some oranges for your children's breakfast this morning. Just let me explain what the problem is. Let's see. How many oranges did you need to make that juice? Three or four. How many mandarins are necessary for the same amount? Seven or eight. When, in your right mind, would you eat three or four oranges for breakfast? Never. When would you be willing to eat seven or eight mandarins at lunch? Never. Are oranges bad? No. Are mandarins the devil? No way!

When you prepare their juice, you and your family are drinking the loose fructose. That fructose goes straight to the liver, and it's a lot. However, you could drink two or three orange or mandarin juices because your brain will never receive the "we're full" signal. Please add up the amount of each of these fruits you would be consuming if you were to drink two glasses.

Let me, therefore, propose a change: why not just eat them? You won't need specialist juicers which cost hundreds of dollars, or blenders with "diamond" blades so that the liquid will turn out just right. Grab them, peel them and straight into your mouth they go. The taste is fantastic. The smell is a marvel. And, by ingesting the pulp, you are certainly ensuring that your beloved orange and darling mandarin are good sources of information for your body. The pulp will give the leptin a heads up and it will then send reliable messages to your brain. Is it that hard? No. But, of course, it means breaking with habit, making a change to your routine, accepting that, for years, you, everyone else and I were squeezing and drinking a lie.

What name could we give to a compound which enters the body, has no benefit for the body and which can only be handled by the liver, the organ responsible for detoxifying the organism? I've got one: poison. Fructose is a poison and it is killing us. It is the main cause of cardiovascular diseases in the world; of diabetes in general, and diabetes in children; of heart attacks in adults and infants; of creating that army of sugar-addicted hunger zombies, of producing anxiety in people and causing dozens more disorders.

God, or the quantum field, or energy, or destiny, or fate, call it what you will, gave us a wonderful gift, fruit, and placed it in perfect doses and filled it with numerous qualities (like fiber). Except Adam, Eve and Snow White, few people have complained about the qualities of *one* apple. But *homo sapiens very sapiens*, in his infinite "wisdom", decided that he was going to alter the form the fruit came in, that it was necessary to drink it and not eat it, that he could convert it into magic powders and add it to all food, including salty, fat-free products —which, due to not having any fat, taste like cardboard and are improved with sugar—. The industry knows this well: the more sugar in their products, the greater an appetite and more of a habit they will generate in their consumers; the "white lady", don't forget, is more addictive than cocaine. And if, on top of this, this way of eating is encouraged by specialists who tell people they need to eat six times a day, the catastrophe will stay right on course. Please, thoroughly check the information on the labels of each product you buy at the supermarket. Please, don't drink juices, and especially not orange or mandarin. Be careful with sugar in all its forms, be it raw sugar cane, honey or syrup, because all of these contain a high proportion of fructose and this is killing humanity. Eat the fruits. Take advantage of their fiber. So what can you drink? I'll tell you later.

Artificial sweeteners

Big industry will always have a solution for everything. When many millions of consumers around the world started to realize what damages sugar caused, the big food and drink companies found a new pretext to keep growing and increasing their worldwide sales: artificial sweeteners. The advertising campaigns, which used slender models, announced the arrival of the age of *light*. No calories. No sucrose. But with the same great taste —or nearly—. Wasn't it great? Artificial sweeteners arrived so that you could consume their products with no guilt attached.

I just want you to remember, while you drink your beverage sweetened with some kind of new substance created in the industry's factories, that all of these sweeteners are derived from chemicals. They are hiding in many foodstuffs under a bunch of different names. The list is gloomy and endless, but I will name some of the usual suspects, like acesulfame, aspartame, maltodextrin, sucralose and... we won't finish this book if I keep naming them.

I put this section directly after the one dedicated to fructose in order to recommend that you don't make the mistake of looking for a replacement for it in the world of artificial sweeteners. That chemical, even if it is in lesser quantities, will also go directly to the liver. And it's a chemical! And it doesn't matter if it contains no calories!

Your organism's metabolic disorders are not prompted by the caloric index; they are caused by the impact that food has on the hormones which regulate your metabolism. All the artificial sweeteners will affect the queen of the hormones, insulin; and some of them will manage to raise her levels ten times more than traditional table sugar. What's more, these chemicals, created by the industry itself, have a greater capability to stimulate your brain centers and activate your eating anxiety and non-stop eating urges. Have you noticed that you are hungrier after drinking a light soft drink or chewing on some gum? Have you noticed that both products contain those magnificent artificial sweeteners?

Each product's commercials and packaging tell us that they are "sugar-free". Very well, but they contain the chemicals we are talking about, which are no good for your organism. Sometimes I notice that people go to a fast-food joint, order an enormous hamburger and, as if to make up for their "sin", they order a light soft drink. Because it's "healthier". I would like to tell all those who follow this habit —hopefully you don't belong to this group— that that drink will raise your insulin in the same way, or even more, than the "regular" or normal soft drink.

"Doctor, you're forgetting something". What? "That there are other natural sweeteners! Those must be good for you". Perhaps you are talking about the so-called *sugar alcohols*, derived from alcohol, such as erythritol, xylitol and maltitol, right? They aren't ideal for your body either. Some studies show that they affect the gut flora. And, at the end of the day, they also raise insulin levels and can increase uric acid levels. I've already told you: if you have elevated insulin levels due to your poor dietary choices, if you generate more uric acid because of an excess of fructose in your diet, and your cortisol is through the roof as a result of a lifestyle which contributes to chronic inflammation, these "three amigos" will start a party inside you which will be very bad for your health.

These chemicals are also found in the infamous protein powders recommended in gyms, and which taste of a Bali piña colada as a result of the chemicals and sweeteners of which it is made up. The label on the tin promises that it does not contain sugar, but if you check in detail it is possible that, among the ingredients of that fabulous tub, you will find maltodextrin (derived from corn), xylitol, sucralose and a lengthy etcetera. But if what you want is to be Mr. Muscle, keep going, show off your magnificent six pack, even if it ends up raising your insulin and uric acid levels.

Avoid artificial sweeteners. When I was wrapping up this chapter, I remembered a very funny song by the Catalan comedians, La Trinca —creators of *I want a busty girlfriend*— called *The light man*, and here is a snippet of the lyrics:

Nothing tastes of what it's supposed to taste of
Nothing contains what it's supposed to contain
Nothing has what it's supposed to have
Nothing is real, everything is so light

Everything is so *light*, and so unhealthy. The message to generation *light* is clear: would you really prefer to consume chemicals than calories? Have you realized that calories are not the cause of your obesity? Do you understand that chemicals are like the detergent you use to wash your clothes? I am going to give you a more alarming example. A few years ago, a group of scientists from Drexel University (United States) discovered that erythritrol, an artificial sweetener, would make a great insecticide. It's no exaggeration, you can find numerous links on the topic online. There is a very nice article in the Spanish newspaper, *ABC*, with the headline: "The sweetener which kills them dead". Enjoy your insecticide.

If you absolutely must sweeten your drinks or food with a calorie-free product, the best option is stevia, and in moderation.

There are those who criticize its bitter aftertaste, but if you use it in smaller quantities it can taste quite pleasant. However, please check that what you are buying is in fact stevia. There are a lot of similar products and some powdered presentations which can be confusing. That's why it is important to read the label. If it says something like "100 % natural sweetener *with* stevia…", leave it right there on the supermarket shelf. You are looking for stevia, not a product "*with* stevia". No doubt if you keep reading the nutrition facts you will discover that it contains erythritol; maltodextrin, 80 %; stevia, 15 %, excipients and other components. That is to say, it is not stevia. It is a near-insecticide sweetener "*with* stevia". Read. Re-read. Check. Don't let them confuse you.

If you are holding *The metabolic miracle* in your hands, it may be because you have discovered that some of your eating habits are not the best for your organism. One of those is the need to sweeten everything. Do you really need to? Your coffee, if you are drinking a good one, does not need sugar; neither do your infusions or your tea. Think about it. It's all about changing your habits, rediscovering flavors, re-educating your body. However, **if the inner monster which has lived with you for so many years is screaming: "Give me sweetness, little one", then go for honey or coconut sugar.** At least you know that they contain 50 % fructose and 50 % glucose, and you already know how they will act inside your organism. The effect of chemicals, on the other hand, can't be known. Better the devil you know. And then, the following day, get back to your sugar-free routine, ok? We can all do it… if we want to.

Supplements

What are dietary supplements? They are nutrients which can usually be found in pill-form, or similar presentations, and which contain a higher dosage than can be found in food in their natural form. Let me give you an example: omega 3. You can find it in certain fish or seaweed, but if you take the supplement (the pill, the capsule, the tablet) you will receive a greater quantity of this valuable fatty acid all at once.

Today they are used all over the world. On a daily basis I prescribe natural supplements such as magnesium, zinc, folic acid, vitamins D and B12, the omega we just spoke about, among others. They are very useful and beneficial to the body if used in moderation, responsibly and only if they are entirely necessary. I tend to use them with my patients in a transitory fashion, while we correct their illnesses. They are very useful, but what I have noticed is that people use them without knowing why.

I often ask those who come into my practice if they take them. Many have given me an affirmative response which surprises me: "Yes, doctor, I have about 15 of those supplements. People bring them over to me from the United States". Almost always, when I check their cases, I conclude that they are taking them unnecessarily. They use them because a friend recommended them or because they are in fashion. This happens a lot with magnesium, which is excellent; studies show that it helps with more than 400 bodily functions, but the benefits of this mineral depend on the salt with which it is mixed. That's why there are sulfates, chlorides, citrates, threonates and many other forms of magnesium. Perhaps the one you need —in the event that you do need it— is different to the one your friend uses. And, obviously, it is best to consult a specialist for guidance.

Many consumers believe that, as they are produced in the land of Trump and approved by the American Food and Drug Administration (FDA), their quality is guaranteed, but that isn't the case. I am telling you this so that you check, please, and read in detail what the ingredients of the supplements you are going to buy are. Pay close attention to the "excipients", which are all the components contained in the tablet and the main molecule. That way you will know what materials were used to make the capsule, to establish if they are from animal or vegetable origin or if they are synthetic. I frequently see poorly manufactured supplements with bad sources, which, in the long-term, can represent a health hazard. Always check, don't forget.

Maybe the supplements which your friends, acquaintances and doctors recommend most are the omegas. They are very good, without doubt, but it is important that you know which one you need. If you buy omega 6 and omega 3, and it turns out that there is an excess of the former in your organism —that would not be odd; as I mentioned earlier, there is an overabundance of it in the world, thanks canola, thanks corn!— and too little of the latter, you will be causing an imbalance. You will raise omega 6 levels even more, but the omega 3 will be beneficial. In conclusion, you only need one; the other one will be useless, it won't help, quite the opposite. It doesn't matter if Aunt Bertha has brought them both over from the United States.

However, omega 3, which is perhaps one of the most consumed supplements, needs to have a specific balance and equilibrium, there needs to be a suitable ratio of EPA (Eicosapentaenoic acid) to DHA (Docosahexaenoic acid), which make it up —remember that omega is a fatty acid—. The ideal ratio should be 3 to 2. If it is different, it is poorly formulated and will not be a beneficial supplement, it will be a "pathological" omega. I have checked these indicators in detail and I can tell you that, according to my observations, only one in every ten omegas is properly formulated. Read the label properly, ask for information. Otherwise you could be buying an unbalanced supplement which will not help your organism. Don't expect miraculous results if you choose the wrong products.

Which omega 3 should you buy? If it's vegetable, make sure it comes from seaweed or linseed oil; if it's animal it should be certified mercury-free and have an EPA/DHA ratio of 3 to 2; otherwise it will not be a good quality supplement.

Another compound which has gained a great many followers is conjugated linoleic acid, known as CLA, which is very trendy in the fitness world as a means to lose weight. This is a good omega 6, found naturally in beef, lamb, duck and turkey, and which additionally has the capability to then convert into omega 3 and provide all of its benefits. It's like a two in one. But... Yes, there is a but: the capsule used for the commonly-prescribed CLA comes from vegetable sources such as soybean, corn and canola, which I have already talked about. On my social media accounts I have covered the issue and I will repeat it here: if you follow a diet which is high in healthy fats and low in carbohydrates you will see very good results in terms of losing weight —if that is your goal—, so why take CLA tablets?

In the midst of this supplement boom, we find licorice. Sometimes consumers buy it without knowing that they did; let me explain: maybe they were looking for a natural energy pill and one of its ingredients is licorice. This, you'll know if you Google it, helps raise cortisol levels, which is the hormone which controls stress. It sounds very logical. If, when faced with the daily worries, you feel downcast and tired, well giving the cortisol a little "push" wouldn't be a bad idea. But it's not good either. I ask you to dip into your memory again. Usually the cortisol measurements taken in the morning for patients who say they are fatigued give misleading results. They almost always reveal low levels of cortisol. But that is because they are producing it at the wrong hours, at night. If the specialist was able to detect it, before recommending licorice they will try to regulate the patient's metabolism so that their cortisol can get its act together. Otherwise, the impetus of the licorice can worsen the panorama. I have seen patients with high blood pressure as a result of excessive use of this supplement. Why? Because if they have elevated cortisol levels, they will no doubt have elevated insulin levels, and with the shot of licorice this will be stimulated further and this will have caused a big mess. Therefore, you should be very careful with its use.

There is another big global trend. Consumers are determined to spend all their money on products referred to as fat "burners". Every day a new one is born which promises something different (which it couldn't possibly achieve). Firstly, there is no external mechanism which "burns" your fat. If there were, if they worked like they claimed to, then all those miraculous girdles advertised on television, or dehydrating yourself for hours in a sauna, would make people thinner; unfortunately, that is not the case. You tell me if you have used therapeutic saunas and have lost weight. I'll believe you. Infrared saunas help reduce the body's inflammation and, therefore, allow you to lose fat, but it isn't a therapy which "burns" lipids and removes spare tires. Am I being clear?

Don't trust those creams which, allegedly, after being applied to your skin, soften or remove fat. No cream can achieve this result. Those fat "burners" which promise to be "thermogenic" —as if raising the body's temperature could help— are a strategy to swindle consumers. To be clear, I should say that there is a real process for burning fat, but it doesn't involve creams, supplements, saunas or telesales, but I'll tell you about it later.

In this burner business, there is a compound on the market which really terrifies me. I won't say its name because it truly is dangerous and it would be irresponsible on my part to even mention it, but I will tell you that it was used in the First World War and it killed lots of people. It was a substance which could be found in bombs, in explosives, and which was present in the warehouses where they were stored, and caused those who were guarding them to suffer intoxication. This element raised their temperature, caused fever in just seconds and, due to the changes in the oxygen intake, they lost weight and then died. The sad thing is that this compound, which was buried for almost a century (and which begins with the letter "d"), has now started to be distributed on the market, with people being given extremely low doses in order to cause "mini-fevers". The next day, those who have taken it will wake up a few kilos lighter, but they are playing with their own lives. Its use seems extremely dangerous and frightening to me.

You will not burn fat if you take a magic pill every day and are still lazing around in front of the television eating donuts like Homer Simpson. A little pill, even if it is the new molecule of the latest molecule of "burner" molecules, will not change your weight, your metabolism, or anything. Control your diet, check what you eat, do exercise, love yourself a little and you will get there.

What can I say about those infamous supplements which they recommend in gyms? Those called something like Ultraboost Macho Man II or Max Energy Plus Reloaded, which promise more strength, more stamina, full energy and greater strenght. Well, that most of them are compounds which do absolutely nothing. Some of them contain amino acids, which are the little building blocks of the structure of proteins. You might say: "Well if, to have muscles like Rambo, you need protein, and these are made up of amino acids, then that tub which gives them to me in a strawberry and vanilla-flavored powder, must be pure gold". But no. Go back a few paragraphs and read about why we shouldn't trust those supplements, with their artificial colors, sweeteners, stabilizers, preservatives and everything else.

Amino acids are very popular. Some people love them, some people hate them. I only recommend them, in vegetable capsules and as a nutritional complement, to those who are training to increase their muscle mass and do not have the adequate gastric functioning. Otherwise there is no point. If you are looking for these results and include a good amount of protein in your diet, you will reach your goal.

Among the cans, jars and different containers made for fitness fanatics you will find a great many which contain sources of protein. The majority of these come from milk and soy whey. Pure protein, zero fat, zero carbohydrates! How do they achieve such a wonder? How do the creators of these powders which turn into shakes with exotic flavors do it, if they are made from "zero"? Marketing and its magic. Again, it's *your* decision; I assure you that you will achieve good muscle mass with appropriate exercise and healthier food sources. Why so many chemicals? Why so many shakes which contain them? Why the excessive consumption of a suspicious protein? Then cancer kicks in and you and your doctor will say that it's your genes, that it was inherited from your grandfather, but you miss the most obvious thing: you gave bad information to your body, you made it sick.

Many of these supplements are killing us. Neither you nor I matter to big industry, what matters is that we buy the supplements and help this big business; and the worst thing is, sadly: many of these products are made with very cheap raw materials and are then sold to us at a high price. It is true that some of these, different ones to those I mentioned, are good and totally necessary —I won't spend time on them here— for supporting the correction of a double illness. But if we are good doctors, good therapists, we can help our patients make their diet the fundamental pillar of their healing, which they won't achieve by means of supplements or a bunch of pills. To fix these disorders, real food is necessary; less fiction, fewer fake shakes. Thomas Alva Edison said it best: "The doctor of the future will not treat illnesses with medication but with food". So welcome to the future.

Dairy products

When we were kids, our parents, pediatricians and television commercials assured us that cow's milk was the best foodstuff in the world. And I agree with that, it is the best foodstuff in the world, but for calves. If you were a calf, you wouldn't be reading this book, no doubt you'd be wandering around, exploring the countryside and then looking for your mother's udder and over time you would become a fully-grown ruminant. But as you are a human being, a valuable member of my pride, you might be interested in the information I am going to give you about this white liquid.

If we look at it from an anthropological viewpoint, if we look at our history, it is evident that we are the only mammal on the planet who, as well as breastfeeding past the lactation period, consumes the milk of another animal out of choice. The vast majority of mammals stop breastfeeding when their teeth come through and their jaw has strengthened. Once they are able to bite and tear solid food, they are ready to change their diet. However, we humans are the rare exception to the rule. We are *really special*.

Everyone in the world should be intolerant to lactose, which is milk sugar. "And why's that, doctor? Have you gone mad?". No, it's a fact. Just as earlier I told you that glucose is a simple sugar —a monosaccharide—, now I'm telling you that lactose is a disaccharide, because its structure is made up of the union of two monosaccharides: glucose and galactose. When we are born, our organism contains a protein called lactase, which is responsible for "breaking up" this disaccharide and separating it into its two components, glucose and galactose. Only thus is our intestine capable of absorbing lactose. That's why babies, in general, don't have any problems feeding off their mother's teat. They are designed to tolerate it.

However, over the years, when their teeth come through, their own development is telling them that the time has come for them to nourish themselves in a different way. Gradually, their organism stops producing lactase. Why would they need it if their breast milk years are over? And on the other hand, it's pretty logical; just like mother cows, goats, giraffes, lions or zebras, human mothers cannot breastfeed their offspring forever. It is a natural evolutionary process. They have other decisive roles to play within their "pride".

But let's get back to the world of people. That baby grows up, turns into a child who has a different diet and their organism starts to forget about that protein, lactase. But for the rest of their life, they will consume lots of dairy products because, as their parents, pediatrician and advertising will tell them, they will help them grow, have stronger bones, avoid osteoporosis and even gastritis. That young person's story (which may seem similar to yours or mine) will be marked by cow's milk. The problem is that their body no longer has that lactase which allows it to absorb the lactose. That's why, when they ingest dairy products, that young person's organism, and then their adult organism, will have to face the challenge alone. But, although their intestine might try, it won't be able to "break up" that disaccharide; it won't be able to absorb that foodstuff from an anonymous bovine. After all, they are a human, not a calf.

If we don't have lactase we will be lactose intolerant. It's that simple. That's why cow's milk derivatives will cause us abdominal inflammation, stomach cramps, pain and even diarrhea, among other symptoms. Is that clear? We are not designed to digest that foodstuff. And here let me make a confession, so that you know that I am on your side. I like dairy products, there must be very few people in the world who do not enjoy a nice cheese, ice cream, pizza, flan; the list is endless. But when I weigh up the pros and cons, I prefer to refrain from consuming them —that doesn't mean that I *never* indulge—.

One hundred percent of humans should be lactose intolerant; however, today's figures show that 30 % of the global population is tolerant to dairy. Three in every ten individuals can absorb them because they keep producing lactase. That is proof that the evolution of the human organism has continued its course, it hasn't stalled —as many scientists claim—. And how ironic, I am one of those 30 %. My body tolerates lactose. Why don't I consume it? Because being able to absorb it or having the capability to break down the lactose and deconstruct it into glucose and galactose is not enough. In the long run, there are many disadvantages of the continued consumption of this disaccharide. Milk is not only sugar, milk contains fat and protein. Don't lose focus, in a couple of paragraphs I will talk about them.

For the time being, I am going to tell you another uncomfortable truth. If you —just like Aunt Bertha— feel healthier and removed from that lactose intolerance mess because you consume lactose-free milk, you are living a lie. When they claim that it is "lactose-free", you are led to believe that they have removed the lactose, but no. What big industry, who created these products, did, is "break it up", dividing it into glucose and galactose so that your body doesn't have to deal with that operation. The disaccharide is therefore separated into two simple sugars. Simple sugars (monosaccharides) have a sweeter taste in the mouth, which is why lactose-free milk is sweeter; you've no doubt noticed. And because of these characteristics, it will be available more quickly in your blood and raise your insulin levels. Therefore, it will fatten you up more than whole milk.

When the age of light products arrived, we took another false step which affected the dairy world. The only good thing that milk and its derivatives contain is their fats, but as the nutrition gods of the United States told the world that these were bad, the industry's companies created their light milk mutations. Dairy products have different types of fat. Just like breast milk, cow, goat and sheep's milk contain a high percentage of good saturated fats and other highly beneficial fats. Perhaps you chose the path signposted by the industry and started to consume dairy products without cream, without fats, lactose-free and you think you did a good thing because you are feeding your body fewer calories —by now you well know that calorie counting is not important— and because you won't suffer lactose intolerance shocks. But no.

The cream or the fat in the yogurt you drank, for example, will have helped make a lower impact on the insulin, but without it, the loose sugar will cause a bigger spike in the hormone.

Most of the "hunger zombies" roaming the supermarkets and buying these lactose-free, skimmed products because they are supposedly light, will, after consuming them for a while, realize that the only "light" thing about all this was their wishful thinking, because those yogurts, creams and milks will make them put on weight and cause metabolic disorders. Don't be part of that clan.

By virtue of repetition, by seeing it on commercials and hearing it on the radio, millions of people believe that it is better to eat those low-fat cheese slices than traditional cheese. But bear in mind that, in order to compact those dairy products which contain no fat, the producers will have to turn to a variety of curdling agents, and some of those contain starches. And what is a starch? Well, another carbohydrate added to the mix, which will end up further activating the insulin of the person consuming it. So, if you are intent on devouring that piece of cheese because the spirit within you is asking for it, then pick a real cheese; it will do you less harm.

Keep in mind, however, that even the taste for cheese has been imposed on us. In the late eighties and early nineties, when dairy companies in the United States started removing the fat from their products, they weren't prepared to lose this residue. So what did they do with those fats? Invent a wide variety of cheeses. That's why, today, we put cheese on everything. They weren't going to lose that money! They never lose, but the consumers do as a result of their ideas.

That's the whey

I have spoken about the sugar in dairy products, about their fats, and now it's the proteins' turn. The preferred choice of those who dedicate their time to the gym, is milk whey. If we only analyze its protein potential, we could say that it has its benefits. But it isn't good for your metabolism because its consumption raises levels of the queen hormone, insulin, too much and too quickly. What would you prefer, protein for your muscles or a disorder in your organism? You choose.

If the best thing about dairy products is their fats, then the worst thing they contain is a protein called casein. Remember that the human intestine works like a strainer: it lets the nutrients it needs through and blocks the entry of the matter which it does not require. Casein leads to the breaking of this organ's cells and causes the so-called intestinal permeability. It creates cracks in the "strainer", messes up its filtration system and allows for the arrival of unwelcome substances.

That's why dairy products are directly linked to multiple illnesses, especially metabolic syndrome: obesity, high blood pressure, high triglycerides, fatty liver, low HDL, and an increase in the abdominal circumference. All of these conditions are the basis for prediabetes, diabetes and chronic vascular problems. What's more, the frequent consumption of cow's milk derivatives is also related to acne and chronic allergies. Let me explain in more detail. Right from the beginning, from the moment a child comes into the world.

Let's suppose that this child is born by cesarean —as is the case with millions of babies today—. As they are not exposed to the maternal birth canal, their gut flora —which is so important— will not be in an ideal state. Maybe the mother of this small child cannot breastfeed and, from their first few weeks of life, they have to drink formula —it happens a lot, more and more frequently—, which means that their contact with casein takes place very shortly after having left the uterus. This milk, which, as well as having that bad protein, also contains lots of sugar, slowly starts to cause damage to the little one's metabolism. That's how their recurring viral infections, rhinitis, conjunctivitis, dermatitis and asthma begin; they will turn into a child with a lot of allergies. Perhaps the family's allergy specialist will tell the parents not to worry, and that "this is hereditary".

But what is really happening is that the little one's intestine is not right. And it can't be right because, from the moment they arrived in their loving parents' arms, they have been consuming casein and sugar. Over time, this child, who then becomes a youth and then an adult, ends up with intestinal impermeability (the broken strainer). That is serious. That needs to be avoided because the intestine is the human body's largest mucus system. The gastrointestinal tract is connected to the respiratory mucus, the skin, the genitourinary system, all of which are interconnected via the lymphatic system. That's why, if there is damage to the intestine, it can manifest itself in the form of allergies in the respiratory system, which are the result of chronic inflammation in the organism. Everything originates from the food that this person has received ever since they were a baby.

There is a very common disease, which affects almost all of us in our teenage years, and that is acne. Decades ago we were told to avoid fats and chocolates, and that that would help to sort it out, if we also applied certain creams recommended to us by the dermatologist. Nobody told us that milk derivatives help to produce it. It's an important topic. The first thing I do to treat acne in my patients is to take dairy products out of their diet and increase their consumption of good fats. "How can you even think that, doctor? Fats cause more spots!", you will no doubt be thinking. However, how odd, what a coincidence, what a miracle, my patients get better. Why? Because the issue of acne is more than skin deep. Yes, there are bacteria which produce it, but I wouldn't recommend prescribing an antibiotic to fight it —that would be sorting out the flooding with mops—. The solution can be found by correcting the metabolic process so that the skin changes and stops being hospitable territory for these bacteria which, with the changed conditions, will no longer be able to spring up there —that is fixing the hole in the ceiling—.

Calcium is another topic. **Aunt Bertha told us for years that we should consume milk because it is rich in calcium, which helps to strengthen our bones. Uncle Pete also said it: "Drink that milk, sonny, so that your bones don't break when you play soccer". They were right** —animal dairy contains calcium, and even vitamin D—, **but their conclusion was wrong. People do not absorb the calcium in cow, sheep or goat's milk!** Our calcium-phosphorous ratio is very different to that of those good quadrupeds. The calcium in cow's milk will be of use to its calf. Breast milk will be of use to a human baby. So, what the dairy industry often does is add calcium to its products so that the *homo sapiens* consumers who buy them in the supermarkets can absorb it. If they don't add it, it won't be of use to us. They add it!

What I just told you isn't just a notion of mine. Many studies show that the countries with the lowest milk consumption rates, like those of East Asia, have the lowest rates of osteoporosis and pathologic fractures from calcium deficiency in the world. "So, doctor, why are we still believing today that we need milk so that our bones don't break?". Because milk is big business. It provides millions of dollars of profit. Everything contains milk! And, what's more, do you know what one of the sponsors of the American Orthopaedic Association has been for years? The United States dairy industry. If orthopaedists, who are the doctors who know most about bones on this planet, recommend that we drink milk so that our tibia or our fibula don't break, well, who is going to contradict them? What they don't tell us is that their studies are not guilt-free because they are backed by the dairy cow industry.

The milky way

Given the evidence, if people want to continue consuming dairy products for life, even though we are missing the lactase in our organism, the most logical thing would be for the primary source to be breast milk, which is made for humans. Right? I know, it seems like a crazy idea. But what is also crazy is this insatiable habit of consuming milk derivatives. Look, if I were to tell you that there is a great company which has started its new business venture using the milk of two million super-healthy human mothers to produce yogurts, ice creams, butters, cheeses and and ultra-pasteurized milk bursting with vitamins, packed in a recyclable, eco-friendly container, and whose sales help the children of the world, you wouldn't buy it, you wouldn't drink it and you wouldn't give it to your kids. Disgusting! But if I change the source of everything I have just mentioned and say that the milk comes from cows, you would consume it. Right? But really, what is more illogical?

The white liquid from those millions of bovine creatures, who no doubt live crowded together in those immense conglomerates where production and quantity come first, passes through a pasteurization process in enormous containers which allegedly eliminate all of the bacteria that the milk might contain. It's true, they do die, but their bacterial DNA stays there and its toxins, lipo-polysaccharides, often remain in the dairy products.

Furthermore, on multiple occasions, the cows have infections, suffer from mastitis and there is pus in their milk. In nations like Australia or New Zealand, there are strict regulations stating that, as well as their vaccinations, the bovine livestock must be injected with a reagent, and in the event that the animal's milk still contains circulating antibiotics, the liquid turns purple and cannot be used. Does the same thing happen in European nations or The Americas? No, at least not in the majority of countries.

Drinking the milk from so many cows, who may have grown up on hormones, which could contain various diseases and pus, ends up causing chronic inflammation in the human consumers, which will then produce all of those organic imbalances that I have already mentioned, which could even have an influence on the development of cancer. Some studies indicate that milk has the capability to increase the so-called insulin-like growth factor, an important cog in the development of carcinogenic diseases.

When I bring up the topic of dairy products, many people share their family anecdotes. "Doctor, my grandfather died at the age of 103 and every day of his life he drank milk, how do you explain that?". Then we start to delve into the story of this century-plus-old man and it turns out that he grew up in the countryside, that he drank the milk from the two or three cows from his farm, grass-fed cows, cows without hormones, real cows. And, what's more, their grandfather had a healthier diet and ate three times a day, never experienced this century's work stresses, was not exposed to so much radiation, did not breathe the air that we put up with. **What affects us is not just consuming dairy products; it's all about how their repeated and sometimes exaggerated consumption, especially in their commercial, sugar-filled or devoid of fat presentations, added to a poor diet, modern-day** stresses, bad habits and sedentarism can lead to the collapse of the entire metabolic scaffold and produce the inevitable destruction of our organism.

We human beings have consumed dairy products for millennia, but not every day. When granddad turned 103 —or the members of the tribes which populated the earth— he drank the milk from his cows, because they had just become pregnant, they had given birth to their offspring and that's why they had it readily available in their body. It was their lactation period. It was temporary. Their udders were not an inexhaustible source of milk. Therefore, it was impossible for granddad —or the Masai tribes of Africa or any other human group— to always have milk handy.

Today, as you know, it is different. Do you want some milk, or lactose-free, light, Queen of the Valley strawberry-flavored yogurt with added cereal chunks? Just go to the supermarket, or order a delivery, and there you have it. The industry constantly has its cows lactating. Their milk is produced thanks to a hormone called prolactin, which is generated by suction, such that, if there are machines suctioning the udders of these ruminants every day, paradise can be attained, we reach the Milky Way.

Crying over spilt milk

This has been a section with a lot of information and maybe a bunch of surprises. I want to end by reminding you of the main ideas on dairy products and giving you some suggestions.

1 › Don't forget that, behind the dietary guides which tell us to consume dairy products, and even some scientific studies which promote their consumption, is the milk derivatives

industry. Trust me: it cares very little about our health, but it does want us to pay for its products.

2 › It is not true that we need milk to make our bones stronger.

3 › Milk is not a good source of calcium for human beings; there are other better sources, such as broccoli, sesame or almonds; in fact, a fistful of the latter could contain up to 10 times more calcium than a glass of milk.

4 › According to some investigations, milk can increase the risk of cancer. There are studies which suggest this, after analyzing several biochemical and immunological factors. But it would be difficult to find an article which clearly states that, which has a good enough number of test patients to demonstrate this, because the dairy industry will deny it and destroy any evidence.

5 › The fat in dairy products does not represent any kind of risk to our organism; the same cannot be said of one of its main proteins, casein, and its sugar, that disaccharide known as lactose.

6 › Dairy products in their lactose-free and fat-free forms, or in their whey protein presentation, can lead the insulin to rise more than it should. Casein and the insulin-like growth factor (IGF-1) can cause chronic inflammation, the root of a list of evils that you should by now be able to name, and even cancer.

"So, doctor, what can I do if I like milk?", you'll ask me, despondently. First of all, relax. I tend to say that the poison is in the dosage and the frequency. I'm sure you'll have heard your smoker friends saying: "I don't have a problem, I only smoke one cigarette a day". Well there's the bad frequency I'm talking about. Or "I hardly smoke any more, but when I do, I smoke every last one". There's the inappropriate consumption. Do you get me?

I know, we live in a world made of milk. And, indeed, its derivatives are really tasty. Here are some suggestions for you to bear in mind, but based on the aforementioned: be careful with the "dosage" and "frequency". If you are going to consume dairy products, first make sure that they are made using whole milk, and ideally that they come from a reliable source. The best thing would be to get them from a farm that you know, with few cows, who are ideally grass-fed and not fed on grains. That would be the best source for your yogurt, cheese, butter or clarified butter (ghee, which is very fashionable right now). That would be the ideal panorama. If that is too hard, then try to find another option which guarantees you a quality product. A trusted organic store or market, for example.

And what about cheese? If you are going to consume cow's milk cheese, it's best to go for a mature cheese which, due to this process of maturing, loses water, dehydrates and some of the proteins within it, like casein, go through a process of denaturation and, above all, what will remain is the fat —which you already know is the best thing about dairy. If I had to choose, I would go for cured goat's and sheep's cheeses, which contain A2 casein— the one in cow's milk is A1—, which, according to some studies, do not cause the harmful effects that cow's milk casein causes in the human body.

There are other forms which could prove to have benefits, like Greek yogurt made with whole milk from a good source —with no added sugar and with all of its fat and cream—, or kefir, that fermented product from the Caucasus which has become very popular. For centuries it has been used as a medicine in the Middle East and it provides probiotic bacteria to the intestine.

But, please, don't consume lactose-free or skimmed milk —I already gave you the reasons— or fat-free cheeses and yogurts, or those dairy products with 'light' on the label, and less still those alleged cheeses that come in a can or a spray. Not for anything in the world! "And what about my strawberry yogurt, doctor? The one they advertise on TV?". No yogurts with added fruits. Don't trust commercials.

If you struggle to resist the "temptation", I propose a solution: take the worst dairy products out of your fridge. No more ice-cream in the freezer. No more sugary yogurts with your cereals —and definitely not for your kids—. No more cheeses in a can. Limit yourself to only good dairy products, like those I mentioned, but regulate their consumption and the amount. And leave the dairy-based desserts for when you go out to eat in a restaurant. That way you will value them and enjoy them more.

Gluten

I'd need a whole other book to talk about this unruly "little guy" who has become a recurring topic in conversations and who triggers heated debates between doctors and nutritionists the world over. Here I will explain, in simple terms, what gluten is and how it acts inside our organism, but if you belong to the radical league of sacred adoring fans of our daily bread, and you resist the belief in the damages it causes, I recommend you follow the studies of pediatric gastroenterologist Alessio Fasano, founder and director of the Center for Celiac Research and Treatment at Massachusetts General Hospital, and author of *Gluten Freedom* (2014), available at your favorite online library. Or, if you're still not satisfied, there is another good text on the subject, written by my professor and neurologist David Perlmutter, called *Grain Brain* (2013). I recommend this reading to complement the general explanations which I will now get into.

With your hand on your heart (and the bread on the table), do you really know what gluten is? It is a protein which makes up part of the lectin group, which are found in wheat, barley and rye. The human body, by the way, isn't particularly fond of lectins. What is really curious is that gluten itself isn't bad, the harmful one is the one we consume today, because it has been genetically modified (like corn, like soybean, remember we covered this topic?).

Thousands of years ago, before man became agricultural, the bread our ancestors ate came from wild wheat. They didn't plant it. It was just there. Then they did grow it, but there was little to fear.

In the last supper, Jesus did not pass around gluten-free bread to his disciples, right? But in the age we live in, that gluten found in wheat, with which the dough for that croissant you had for breakfast and will no doubt eat tomorrow and the rest of the week was made, is a mutation. That mutation, that Transformer lectin, is entering your body all-too-frequently.

"But what does gluten do the body, doctor?". Oh, hardly anything: it just causes intestinal permeability, which we have spoken about in various sections of *The metabolic miracle*. The intestine is a strainer. It lets in the "good" stuff and blocks the "bad" stuff. Gluten breaks that strainer and messes up this filtration job. Doctor Fasano has described, in detail, all the structural physiological, biochemical and immunological damage done to the intestinal barrier as a result of this lectin. At the beginning of this century, alongside his team of scientists, this doctor discovered a molecule called zonulin, which carries out a very important role in the intestinal cells' sieve work. The zonulin lets them know whether to allow a certain substance to pass through. The trouble arises when, due to some disorder, the zonulin gives the wrong instructions and makes the cells open their doors at unsuitable times and for longer than they should. I won't go into more detail, I don't want to digress from my objective, which is to tell you all this in the simplest possible terms, but Alessio Fanaso's findings are fascinating.

So, the strainer is broken. The gluten begins to generate a localized chronic inflammation in your body. The intestine cannot block the arrival of "enemies". Through its gateway cells flood tons of fungi, bacteria, parasites; on noticing the presence of these undesired guests, your immune system will want to go to war, and the way it conducts combat is to generate an inflammatory response, which will be constant, as the enemies will keep coming through the breached intestine. It's like an endless battle between the police (the immune system) and the criminals (the unwelcome bacteria or substances).

Through different paths, the ferocious gluten from your beloved bread produces chronic conditions such as allergies, diabetes, and chronic gastrointestinal problems, but it can also be the creator of autoimmune diseases like lupus, rheumatoid arthritis, Sjögren's syndrome, type 1 diabetes, Lou Gehrig's disease, multiple sclerosis and various forms of cancer: breast, prostate, colon, pancreatic, intestinal, among others.

Who are those affected by this wheat protein? All consumers, but there are specific cases. On the one hand we find those who suffer from celiac disease, which means their body cannot tolerate said lectin and, faced with its arrival, their intestine produces a very severe reaction, with similar symptoms to those seen in lactose intolerant people: a lot of gas, strong stomach pains, sharp cramps, and sometimes explosive diarrhea. The bulk of the population affected by gluten does not suffer such obvious discomfort because it is made up of people who have "sensitivity". In many cases they do not even present gastrointestinal pain and the symptoms can become apparent up to 72 hours after exposure to the wheat protein. Sometimes their sensitivity manifests itself in their skin or in mental episodes; I have seen cases of people who suffer hallucinations two days after consuming some food which contains gluten. That's why it is often difficult for doctors to identify those cases of sensitivity, because the discomfort in patients arises many hours after the food has been ingested.

Gluten is, without doubt, one of the great scourges of the modern, industrial age, due to the damage caused and the consequences. It's not just in your bread in the morning; it is in pasta, cookies, tortillas, toast. Take note: there are even soy sauce brands which include it. Some time ago, reading the ingredients of one of them in the supermarket, I found that the three main ingredients, from greatest proportion to smallest proportion, were water, wheat and soybean. So why don't they call it "gluten sauce"? Thoroughly check the labels of what you are planning on buying. And be very aware, too, that buying oats or oat flour —both of which are very good— to make your waffles or pancakes is of no use if they are not certified products. Often wheat flour —the gluten-filled cousin— is stored alongside oat flour— the gluten-free cousin— and contaminates it.

I have nothing against bread or products made using wheat. They are delicious. But if you and I analyze them, if we place their pros and cons on scales, the latter will be heavier. Gluten will induce chronic inflammation in our body, which marks the beginning of the path towards many chronic diseases and metabolic syndrome. **So here is my advice: if you are a celiac, avoid gluten; if you are sensitive to gluten, avoid it; if you are not a celiac and you are not gluten sensitive, avoid it too. "What are you saying, doctor?". Exactly what you read, avoid it! Or limit its consumption to a minimum, unless you want your beloved intestine to end up like a broken strainer.**

"So, doctor, I should only buy gluten-free products?". As I got to the end of this chapter, I was thinking about the efforts we humans have made to create falsely healthy alternatives to all of those foods which can make us sick. To replace sugar they made artificial sweeteners. To "simulate" dairy products they invented the lactose-free versions. And then there are the light and fat-free mutations. And, why not the latest trend: gluten-free baked goods! Which, on top of it all, have an army of influencers recommending them on social media. It is true that some of the options that this gluten-free bakery world offers can be healthy. However, from a metabolic point of view, these breads behave in the same way as others, and you will just end up with gluten-free chubbiness or spare tires.

There are some recipes and products which will help you to correct your intestinal permeability, including aloe vera, stock made with chicken or fish bones —prepared over a low heat— and glutamine powder, which is often used in the sporting world for muscle recovery.

I love the fish bone stock option, but it isn't that easy to prepare. So, if you want to make a simple drink which contributes to the cause, I have just the recipe for you: take a piece of aloe vera crystals, blend it in water with half a squeezed lemon and, when the mixture takes on the appearance of a consistent, frothy lemonade, that is the moment to drink it. This will prove beneficial to your gastric health and crucial to reversing the damage done by gluten. Cheers!

Chapter 7

Physical activity

Working out on an empty stomach

As I mentioned a few chapters ago, I like exercise and I tend to do it very early in the morning, when the city is still asleep and before getting to my practice. It was precisely on one of those early mornings that I was thinking about how to explain to you the importance of this section of the book. I think the most direct way to do it is just to tell you that this is valuable information, that you should pay close attention to the following lines and that, yes, of course it is ok to do sports without having eaten breakfast. Let me explain.

Once again, let's debunk certain myths: a) you won't die if you go for a jog, do your weights routine or take on your cardio session on an empty stomach; b) you won't burn your own muscle; c) if you do it responsibly, your body will thank you. A few pages back, I explained in what order our organism uses the energy it has collected from the information (food) we have given it. First your body will consume the energy from the glucose which is stored in the liver, this is the source we have the most rapid access to. Second, when this runs out, your organism turns to the energy reserves that you have stored in the form of fat —by the process called gluconeogenesis or new creation of glucose— and, third, yes, your body will resort to the protein, but this does not necessarily come from your muscle; its origin could be the skin proteins, which you will have in excess when you lose weight —I will develop this further towards the end of the chapter—. I repeat, your muscle won't be destroyed or "devoured", nor will you end up in intensive care.

Working out on an empty stomach will allow you to do what is promised on telesales channels: burn your fat! Really, no tricks, no ploys. Let's say you had dinner at 7:00 in the evening —by the way, try not to have dinner too late—. And you didn't eat anything else because, following the traditions of your wise grandparents, that was your third meal of the day and that was enough. Therefore, from that point your insulin would be "chilled out". Throughout the night, while you sleep, your body will be consuming the glucose levels in your liver. If you wake up at 5:00 or 6:00 in the morning the next day and go to work out, you will still have a bit of glycogen in your liver and you will be using the energy stored in that organ; that will be the energy you use to exercise, and, sure, you will really "burn" it; I know that you like that verb. When this resource runs out, you will begin to consume your own fat, which will be the energy source used to keep going and not "burn out". That is the way to do it, which is a little different from what Aunt Bertha told you, which was to drink some hot water with lemon on an empty stomach, "so that you burn that fat, kiddo".

"But, doctor, if I go out jogging without having breakfast, or eating my energy bars or drinking my protein shake, I might get dizzy", you might say out loud. You won't get "dizzy", don't worry. Look, I have been a high performance athlete for many

years now; I have run marathons on an empty stomach on numerous occasions and here I am, writing this, still alive. And I never got "dizzy"! Let me give you an example. When you go out for dinner with your partner, you carry a certain amount of money in your wallet. Even if your personal wealth was greater than that of Jeff Bezos, you wouldn't be able to have much cash in it, because your wallet has a limit, right? Whatever fits, fits. So dinner was spectacular and you pay with all your cash. But your partner suggests you go out on the town (clubbing, on a blow-out, painting the town red, whatever you want to call it) and, as you no longer have cash on you but your bank account contains sufficient funds to party all night long, you pay with your credit card.

Now imagine that the wallet is your liver and the cash is the glycogen stored within. Only a certain amount of glycogen —cash, dough— fits in the organ and what is left over is exported from the liver in the form of fat, which you accumulate in your various organs or tissues, and this is what forms the so-called spare tires. This fat is like the money you have in your bank account —which doesn't fit in your wallet. It's there, safe, ready to be used—. If you go out jogging on an empty stomach your organism won't be able to make use of the "rapid energy", the cash, because most of it was used up during the night —you might have a little left—; however, that's what the fat is there for, it is like the funds saved in your bank account, so use your credit or debit cards without any worries. Go out to train, knowing that you are using up the energy in your fat, that you have sufficient funds to do it. And spend! You'll have money (energy) left over and it'll do you good.

You've spent the cash in your liver, used up your fat bank savings; and what happens when the latter run out— if that ever happens? Well you'll have to make use of your properties, your protein assets. But you won't "consume" your muscle, I assure you, and that won't happen because your organism is very wise and, when you are deprived of food, it produces a growth hormone which will protect your muscle system. There is no way it is going to provoke the destruction of your muscles.

When we fast, remnants of protein are found in our blood, but these do not come from our muscle, they come from our skin. What do you mean? Let's clear this up, we had it pending. If we put on weight, we will experience an increase in fat and skin. But the cellular growth of each is different. Fat cells increase in size infinitely —this is a process called hypertrophy—, but they do not increase in quantity. Skin cells do not grow or stretch, but they do multiply —this is known as hyperplasia—. That's why, for example, pregnant women get stretch marks, because the increase in the size of the body, which contains the fetus, is quicker than the skin cells' capability to multiply, and as these do not stretch like fat cells, they break and form the marks.

If you train this way, you will lose weight, and with this weight loss you will begin to correct your metabolism. But I am not proposing a weight loss routine, what I am proposing is that you start your metabolic change, your own way of healing yourself. If you work out on an empty stomach, the lipids contained in your fat cells are going to leave them because you are using them as energy. Meanwhile, as far as the skin cells are concerned, there will be staff cutbacks, because, if your bodily dimensions are decreasing, you will have less skin.

Let's get back to pregnant women. When they give birth, that skin which was tensed for months due to the high abdominal content will lose its shape, become flaccid for a few months and then get its shape back. The same thing will happen when someone is losing weight; they no longer need so much skin, so there needs to be a lowering of the number of cells which make it up. Many of these will be fired from their job; this process is known as autophagy, or the capability of the human body to "eat" itself. We will discuss this in detail at the end of *The metabolic miracle.*

I have told you all this in order to explain that, if you work out without eating breakfast and there are proteins in your bloodstream, this will not have come from you muscles, but from that skin which, faced with your physical changes, is reducing its number of employees. Are you now making sense of it?

Training on an empty stomach has many benefits for your metabolism, because it helps to control the queen hormone, insulin; it allows you to rapidly access your fat as a source of energy —this is your bank savings— and assists in the production of growth hormones.

"But doctor, without breakfast I will get dizzy, I assure you", you will repeat. Try it out. If you experience some kind of problem when exercising this way it is because you must have high insulin levels, which is why your sugar levels drop when you train. This is, without doubt, a sign that your metabolism is not right. An organism free of metabolic disorders is capable of exercising in the morning without the help of energy bars or chemical-filled vanilla shakes. What's more, there is another advantage: if you do sports without eating beforehand you will be free of any kind of bloated feeling.

"Doctor, I can only exercise at night, what should I do?". In that case I recommend that you have dinner before training. After dinner, your body will make the last insulin spike, and when you go out to carry out your routine you will be consuming the rapid energy that comes from the glycogen stored in your liver. Afterwards, as you will *not* eat any more —this is important—, towards the end of the night or early in the morning, you will access the energy provided by your own body fat. If you can choose your form of exercise, the first one is ideal, in the morning and on an empty stomach —that way you will have the hormonal assistance of cortisol and insulin—. Do it, you will notice the change.

The greatest desire of half of humanity is to "burn" their body fat. And you can, in a very easy and friendly fashion. I laid it out for you here, it involves using those fat reserves as your main engine; they are an abundant, appropriate, good and pleasant energy source for the body. Let me give you another example. There are numerous ways to light a fire. If you want a quick fire, you can use a bunch of newspaper; as you bring the lighter flame near, there will immediately be fire, but how long will it last? If you have a bit more patience, you will opt for wood, which takes a little longer to catch fire, but will give you lasting fire and heat. Each person chooses which type of fire they need to switch on their body's engine. If you opt for carbohydrate, you will have chosen the newspaper. If, on the other hand, you learn to use your own fat, you will have plenty of good wood.

And, for the love of God, forget about girdles, fat-reducing gels or the miracle burner, and begin your own fat "burning" routines using the correct physiological and biochemical mechanisms. You can make the miracle happen!

Cardio or weights?

Both. Both practices are very good and each person, depending on the results they are looking for, can choose the one which suits them best. I don't intend to tell you which is better, neither is "better". It's not about a competition between long-distance runners and gym lovers. I am going to give you some suggestions for how each one of these practices can help our metabolism.

If you have decided to go for a cardiovascular ("cardio") routine in order to recover the proper functioning of your metabolism, the best advice would be to avoid low-intensity cardio sessions, that is to say those which take place over a longer period of time, but which involve a constant speed or intensity, without large changes, like riding a bike or jogging. If you're looking to get your metabolic framework in order, I suggest you follow the renowned *HIIT*, or high-intensity interval training, routine. In a nutshell, it involves very intense 3 to 5 minute exercises, followed by a minute of low-intensity exercises. This change of rhythm will generate variations in your heart rate and can help your body reach the process of "keto-adaptation" and improve its oxygen consumption. At the end of the day, this is the true definition of metabolism.

Keto-adaptation is, simply put, that mechanism which is set in motion with exercise on an empty stomach. It is the way that your body rapidly consumes glycogen in order to make use of its own fat as a source of energy. Oh, by the way, this is important: keto-adaptation is different to ketosis, which we talked about in the section on fats. Although it sounds like a tongue-twister, all patients in ketosis are keto-adapted. But you can also reach keto-adaptation in other ways. If, as well as being interested in fitness metabolism, you are a keen reader, I recommend that you check out the bibliographic references on the previous chapter (which are at the end of this book). Feast on the banquet and understand, in depth, the biochemistry and physiology behind keto-adaptation —as well as its bountiful benefits—.

On the other side of the coin from cardio is weight training. This practice is carried out in order to achieve three basic goals: 1) to generate muscle mass, hypertrophy; 2) to build strength; 3) to build up resistance. This type of training tends to throw up two opposing figures: the super-muscular Arnold "Terminator" Schwarzenegger-esque sportsman, and the slim person with defined muscles, like a soldier in training. The former is just a lump, they have worked out to gain muscle, but this hypertrophy does not mean that they are particularly strong. I have seen numerous sportsmen with these characteristics who, at the end of the day, have trouble picking up a mattress during a move. The latter, at first glance, just looks like a regular person, skinny, without much strength, but they take off their top in the park and do 300 push-ups on the tips of their fingers in 30 seconds. They have tremendous resistance.

If you choose weightlifting aimed at hypertrophy, your oxygen consumption will make the use of your own fat as an energy source very efficient, especially if you do it on an empty stomach in the morning. There are also some amusing myths surrounding this practice. People tend to say that, if you lift weights, the fat in your body will harden. False! Those with "hard" fat in their organism have some kind of disorder in their metabolism, caused by the hormones I introduced at the beginning of this book. In fact, it has been proven that weight lifting is one of the practices which is most helpful for weight loss.

Another benefit of lifting weights on an empty stomach is that is will naturally produce the growth hormone, which is crucial to good bodily development. Our body has two natural ways of stimulating said hormone: ketosis and fasting. The former is a very useful mechanism for facing conditions like cancer or neurodegenerative diseases like Alzheimer's and Parkinson's (I already mentioned this). Fasting, for its part, and although it seems strange, has helped hundreds of body-builders put on weight, using this healthy and natural means of creating the growth hormone. They thus avoid synthetic hormone injections which can cause tumors.

By the way, the actor Hugh Jackman, star of *The Wolverine* (2013) and the X-Men saga, sculpted that muscular body which appears in the movies by reducing fat through fasting and building muscle mass by exercising on an empty stomach in order to naturally produce the growth hormone.

After reading these paragraphs, what conclusions will you draw? Weights or cardio? My suggestion would be that, on the days that you lift weights, you do very little cardio —just enough to warm up—. Ideally your routine should include the so-called compound exercises, which are better than the isolation exercises.

That way you will work out more muscles in one go. Do the ones you like, but these are my favorites if you want to try them out —if you're not interested in these routines, just skip to the next paragraph—. I do them in different routines, four times a week. I do a flat, decline bench press with dumbbells or a bar; the military press, always in front of my head, the deadlift, dips; pull-ups (using a bar) with a pronated grip (hands facing forward); row, with barbell or dumbbells; free squat or Smith machine squat; the Bulgarian split squat, and supinated pull-ups for the biceps.

And for those days you are doing your cardiovascular routines, follow the high-intensity interval training. **I therefore recommend that you combine these practices. They both have their benefits. The first will help develop your body's muscles, while the second will be very beneficial to your circulation. Complementing both will help with your metabolic balance.** If you lift weights on Monday, Wednesday and Friday, do your cardio on Tuesday and Thursday. And always on an empty stomach.

Lastly, after working out, you do not have to hurriedly pounce like a lion in full hunt on all the protein you can get your hands on. Studies show that a protein intake is effective up to five hours after a sporting activity. Try it; it will also help you recover your metabolic order.

It has been proven that one of the main factors in achieving a suitable metabolism and contributing to its longevity and positive vitality is having good muscle mass. This is achieved by training right, but also by eating right. Without getting caught up in unnecessary protein orgies! If you combine the two variables you will have a well-defined body, as a result of an interior in harmony and thanks to a suitable complementary diet.

Sleep little, train a lot...

Read the title of this section carefully. Read it again, please. Do you think that sleeping little and training a lot makes sense? I just ask because thousands of people believe that this is the best way to lose weight, but I don't think that this combination helps at all. Sleeping is very important for your organism and for your metabolism to be right. During sleep hours, you release a hormone called melatonin. This, as well as "switching off your hard drive" or helping your body to remain in "sleep mode", also has very powerful antioxidant properties. If you don't sleep enough, you won't produce enough melatonin and oxytocin, and will therefore have an imbalance between your antioxidants and the free radicals —I introduced them to you in the chapter on chronic inflammation—.

So what will happen? At night you will have elevated cortisol —the hormone which keeps you alert— levels and, therefore, in the morning you will feel exhausted and your body will enter a fatigue cycle which you provoked. Don't forget what happens when cortisol, insulin, uric acid and leptin get together... This could cause serious metabolic imbalances and, in summary, you will put on weight. And what will you do when you gain weight? Up your dosage of exercise. You will go all out in the gym and that won't help either.

Overtraining will make you produce even more cortisol. Why? Because you are "stressing" your organism out. Therefore, don't play with fire. Sleep well —that really is an important exercise— and find the time to train. I know that, these days, we have very long work days, and work doesn't leave us the time to do anything, but we can always find moments for sleep and exercise. What's more, if you really want a sculpted body, you should know that sleeping well is one of the most crucial factors for proper muscle recovery and repair.

Confess your sins and be forgiven...

My patients ask me all the time: "Can I commit a sin, doctor?". They are talking about food, obviously. "Can I eat a dessert full of calories, sugar, gluten and dairy, from time to time?". Here we go again. Calories are not a problem. Sugar and gluten and dairy are. However, remember that we spoke about how the "quantity" and "frequency" with which you consume them play a big part. **To sum up: yes, of course, eat your dessert now and then. Now and then! I also do it, don't think that I am a lettuce-only martyr. But then get back to your good eating habits. The important thing is maintaining the balance.**

In the cool jargon of the 21st century, this is called a *cheat meal*, cheating a little bit on your diet. If you feel like eating a dessert, first make sure that it is the one you want, the one you crave, one which is worth it; not a cheap option —I'm not talking about the price, but about the ingredients—. If you want a chocolate fondant with old style vanilla ice cream, then go to the place which makes the one to take your breath away. Enjoy it, don't blame yourself for that moment of pleasure. Don't transfer feelings of guilt to your food, be thankful that you can eat it.

Don't look for a light dessert. It's nonsense: the taste won't be what you are hoping for, but the guilt of eating it will be the same. What's more, you know very well by now that artificial sweeteners affect the metabolism in the same way or more than sugar, and that gluten-free or fat-free flours are no guarantee. There are very famous ice-cream shops which sell "diet" or "suitable for diabetics" ice-creams because they are sweetened with pure fructose. Yes, you read that correctly. What an atrocity! You stay away from them. They are pure poison.

Why am I talking about this in the "Physical activity" section? Because when you feel guilty for going off script, for having that cheat meal, for cheating on your diet, you'll no doubt want to make a beeline for the gym or spend three hours running in the park to "kill" the calories you ate. That way you will feel less guilt. "But doctor, I can repent for my sins", a lot of people tell me. Hmm... No, it doesn't work like that. I'm not going to repeat my discourse again, I don't want to bore you, so go back to the section entitled "The big lie....", where all is explained. **Our body doesn't operate on caloric arithmetic; movement, dancing or exercise are not enough to make up for that tiramisu which you ate with so much pleasure (tell that to the Obamas). You didn't "cheat" on your diet. You knew what you were doing, you wanted it, you enjoyed it, that dessert was great, no regrets. Tomorrow get back to your healthy routine, and that's it. Leave the melodrama to the soap operas.**

Two more things before finishing this section. A poor diet could never be made up for with three centuries of exercise. There is no "formula" called "eat badly and then make up for it by training". You can't. It can't be done.

And forget the famous IIFYM (*If It Fits Your Macros*) diet, which I also mentioned already, and which only takes into account the percentage of daily macronutrients you take in, but not which ones these should be.

If the diet says that 35 or 40 % of the calories in your food should come from carbohydrates, don't just focus on the figures; remember that eating a "*pain au chocolat*" is not the same as eating a serving of broccoli, even if the two sources provide the same amount of carb calories.

Elsewhere, there has been an increase in the power of the voices of those on social media who, despite not having studied the workings of the human body in detail, speak about "flexible dieting", which simply promotes the fact that we are in caloric deficit, and that we should add, subtract, multiply and divide calories and "macros" (macronutrients). Do I need to say it again? This math does not work with our metabolism. This cheap tactic may help lots of people look really great on the outside, but they are very sick on the inside. Don't be one of those people.

I am going to use my older brother as an example (I hope he doesn't kill me for this), who tends to say that our organism will be fine if we eat "anything" but "in moderation". It sounds logical, but his assessment is flawed. Firstly, what is eating "anything"? What would the dietary model look like? Secondly, what is moderation? At the end of the day, my dear brother's diet could look like this: two juices, a cookie, a coffee with a teaspoon of brown sugar, a tortilla for his wrap at lunchtime, a flavored water with sweetener, fifteen almonds fried in canola oil, half a light yogurt made with lactose-free milk and the granola that a yogi friend gave him. That is not a flexible diet! That would be a sort of semi-Tibetan diet with which the honorable Dalai Lama would accept an invitation to our house. That model doesn't work.

Agreed? I'll be able to sleep easy if I know that what I have told you is clear. It's all about living a full life, with consistency, and giving ourselves occasional permission to indulge (in a delicious chocolate cake), and that those moments make us sparkle.

Chapter 8

False collective beliefs

"Eating at the wrong times makes you fat"

In this section of the book, I want to debunk some more beliefs about our eating habits, which, as a result of mere repetition, have become supposed truths, even though they are clearly not. Let's start with the jewel in the crown, a recurring phrase from Aunt Bertha: "My boy, if you eat at the wrong times, you will get fat". Relax, Auntie, that's not going to happen.

Remember that the hormone which makes all of us fat is insulin. That is proven and we have spoken extensively about it here —just look at the weight increase on those who have to inject it—. So, obesity is not a consequence of eating at the wrong times, it is the result of overstimulation of our insulin and not letting it rest enough.

"But doctor, you need to eat at a fixed time!", you'll be telling me. Don't be so strict. I recommend the following. It will give good results. Every day, try to feed yourself within a 12-hour window, so that, if you have breakfast at 7:00 in the morning, you should ideally have dinner at 7:00 at night and, from that moment on, mouth shut: let your body rest and don't make the insulin work overtime. You won't die of starvation.

Within those twelve hours, I recommend that you eat three times a day, maximum, and follow the instructions I have laid out in this book. Those three moments of sitting at the table will be enough for your organism to be ok; and it's a habit that fits in with the rhythm of modern life, but there is no divine order carved in stone which lays out the obligatory number of daily meals, because it could be fewer than three —but never more—. Try, if possible, to leave a period of five hours' rest between each meal. For example, have breakfast at 7:00 in the morning, lunch at 1:00 in the afternoon and dinner at 7:00 in the evening.

But, from a physiological point of view, nothing is going to happen to your organism if, one day, you have breakfast at 9:00 in the morning, lunch at 3:00 in the afternoon and dinner at 8:00 in the evening (and if you don't change those times every day). The important thing is to respect that 12-hour window. That will ensure that your insulin is very happy, because it gets to work at the rhythm which suits it. And if your insulin is happy, your metabolism will also be happy and you will be a veritable ocean of bliss. But if you have breakfast at 6:00 in the morning, eat a mid-morning snack at 9:00, have lunch at 1:00 in the afternoon, go for an afternoon dessert at 3:00, have dinner at 6:00 in the evening, have another "mini-dinner" three hours later and then drink a glass of milk with a chocolate cookie at 10:30 at night, while you watch Netflix, well, what a mess! Your insulin will constantly be working and… you already know that whole glucose process in your body off by heart.

My message is this: eat three times a day within a 12-hour window, and give your body the next 12-hour period for its

valuable fast. **Preferably leave a five-hour gap between each meal, so as not to cause unexpected "spikes" in your insulin. Don't panic if you can't have breakfast, lunch and dinner at the same exact time every day.** If you respect this time margin, have a base of healthy carbohydrates and the appropriate percentage of good proteins and fats when you eat, you won't put on weight, even if you eat at the wrong time. Obviously, don't let it become a habit. Next!

"Children need something sweet"

No, children need us, as parents, to teach them how to eat right. Why did this idea that we have to give our children sweets all the time become so popular? Because old scientific theories and the food industry reinforced the idea that, hidden in the paradise of candy, breakfast cereals, chocolate milks, jelly candy and soft drinks, was the energy of life. It is true that glucose provides energy to our cells and helps our body work, but, as we have seen, there are other energy sources. Sweets, which are carbohydrates, are the cheapest and least long-lasting energy source we can access.

That phrase "children need something sweet" is, no doubt, from the makers of "I'm going to eat some chocolate because I'm cold". **There is something I don't understand: if sugar (or sucrose) is one of the most addictive substances on the planet, if its combination of 50 % glucose and 50 % fructose causes millions of deaths around the world, why would it be good for minors?** In my practice I have seen to eight year-old children who have suffered heart attacks or who have diabetes or prediabetes. Every day I see more young people with high blood pressure or cerebral thrombosis, diseases which were previously only seen in adults or the elderly.

And what is the cause of their illnesses? Their prolonged consumption of this supposed "energy of life". A child with a high level of sugar consumption has a 100 % chance of developing metabolic disorders and becoming a sick adult. That is the current reality. Have you noticed that a tub of stage two formula for babies contains a pound of added sugar? And they will drink five bottles a day! We are creating little sugar addicts.

I often ask my adult patients who are looking for a solution to their metabolic disorder which started in childhood if they would have liked their parents to have told them about the risks of sucrose when they were growing up. All of them say yes. But we human beings are full of contradictions. When some of these patients bring me their small children to start to change their eating habits, they are suddenly hit with the feeling of guilt. They feel like bad parents because they have to face social criticism; other people will tell them not to exaggerate, that sweets go hand in hand with kids. Because of this, if sugar is an essential part of childhood, then disease will be an essential part of adulthood. This does not mean that your child should forget about ice-cream or desserts, this is just a call for you to thoroughly examine their diet and how much sugar is included in it (quantity and frequency, remember?).

Teaching children is very easy. They are the best patients. They understand everything better than we do. After a couple of tantrums, they will have changed their diet, just like that. The problem with small children is their parents. Up until the age of eight, children generally have their parents' conscience. If their mother has eating anxiety for sweets, for example, the child will acquire the same custom, but if she changes her habits, her child will too. Obviously a good paternal example is also vital, but during those years the child will more closely follow the behavioral patterns of the person who had them inside her. The important thing is for both mom and dad to have sincerely accepted the change. The effort will be worth nothing if, when the child isn't looking, his parents sneak off to the closet to eat a packet of vanilla cookies on the sly. We are our children's conscience. If we make good dietary decisions, so will they.

My most beautiful moments as a functional doctor have come when I realize that my little patients have learnt to heal themselves. Seeing a girl or boy of seven or eight years-old totally convinced by their healthy eating model —far removed from chip packets and the sweet poison— is incredibly moving. What's more, every little one who makes this decision will act as an example to their friends, who will surely learn from them.

Change begins with us and our example. No more rewarding our children by taking them to a junk food restaurant to enjoy a "banquet". Or filling them up with chocolates that do not even contain cacao, or with jelly sweets and packets of multi-colored candy —with their various chemicals—. Is that really a reward? Of course not.

"Skinny people can eat whatever they like because they don't get fat"

It is often believed that skinny people are very healthy and lucky to boot. Firstly, due to divine intervention: "God made him skinny"; secondly, because, as Aunt Bertha would say, "skinny people have fast metabolism". On the other side of the coin, and following on from the same logic, those who put on weight quickly and suffer from obesity "are being punished by God" and, in the words our dear auntie, "fat people have slow metabolism. But there's nothing they can do about it, it's genetic, dear boy!". Ok. This whole paragraph is a lie.

Being skinny isn't a blessing, and being fat isn't a curse. And, with regards to inherited traits, remember that, according to epigenetics, we can all change the genetic story we receive as a family hand-me-down. It is entirely false that skinny people are healthier and that they can eat what they like. Around the world, the number of thin people suffering from heart attacks, diabetes, fatty liver, high cholesterol and even cerebral thrombosis has risen. Why, if he is skinny and appears to be "healthy", does he have health problems? The answer to this question began to reveal itself through the analysis of various diagnostic images. With these, radiologists discovered that many skinny patients had an infiltration of fat in their livers and that they had started to generate fat around their organs. These are the defining characteristics of *TOFI* (Thin on the Outside, Fat on the Inside) people, or those universally known as metabolically obese normal-weight individuals.

It is very common to find it. But sometimes it is hard to find the cause of their malady because their appearance is misleading. From a clinical point of view, I prefer to attend to people who eat really badly and have put on weight. The evidence is clear and over time we can recover the proper working of their metabolism and their appropriate weight. But with skinny patients who do not put on weight despite eating terribly, or those who are overweight —and can't lose it— despite having very healthy habits, sometimes it is hard to find the "leak". The latter behave like a dam (we have to understand what the blockage is which does not allow their body to drop even a single gram), while the former, due to their appearance, have a disguise. The body of the skinny person, paradoxically, hides their "fat" problem.

So, **if you are a thin woman or a skinny man, but you have some symptoms or problems in your body, like those you have read about in the pages of this book, go to a specialist to have your metabolism checked out. Your skinniness is no protection, it is not a guarantee of health; maybe your illness is hiding behind a curtain and you are under the illusion that you are healthy when you are not.** What's your diet like? Are you sleeping well? Do you exercise? Do you feed your mind and your spirit? Check yourself out: what the scales show is just a figure which could be hiding something.

"You need will power to eat right"

Maybe this happens. After having a breakfast of four pancakes with butter, maple syrup, jelly, two fried eggs with bacon and two mugs of bad coffee with sugar, you take a look in the mirror, notice you are overweight again and feel incredibly annoyed because, once again, you didn't have that "will power" to control your appetite, begin to feed yourself differently and take the first step towards a new life. Despite your annoyance, the servings of your lunch will be equally abundant and wrong. Dinner will be a similar disaster. You want to change, but you can't gather the "power". And you feel distressed for that reason and the distress turns into anxiety, and the anxiety makes you hungry. And you will eat more than you should. Well, this whole section is written just for you.

I have several things to say to you: 1) millions of people on Planet Earth feel the same way as you; 2) of course you can gather that will power to rewrite your story; 3) don't blame yourself, no doubt your metabolism is so unsettled that it does not allow you to think and act clearly, despite your will to change. The fundamental thing is this: that you really *do* want to take that step towards a better way of feeding yourself. Do you?

With everything you have read up until now, you have enough tools to know if there is a metabolic disorder inside you. It's in the curves in your figure, the products in your fridge and cupboard, the number of times you eat a day, the amount of time you dedicate to yourself to give yourself a real *like* for doing something really good, in particular the number of hours you have slept, or dedicated to an exercise routine, or which you have used to punish yourself for "sinning" with so much dessert. If your metabolism is off, if you're hormones are having a party, if the insulin has got together with leptin, cortisol and uric acid, among other pals, then you are no doubt eating this way because you have lost control of your actions. Let's say that the diabolical spirit, Hunger (who we have spoken about), has possessed you. You cannot control your appetite.

It is even more complicated because eating does not have a reward mechanism and generates guilt, like many other addictions. Today, addiction to food is the most common addiction in the world, but nobody wants to accept it. We have become addicted to it, with the help of the false prophets of nutrition who tell us that we need to eat six times a day, which creates a conditioned neurohormonal response, like Pavlov's dogs. And big industry gives us another shove towards addiction by adding unnecessary elements (like sugar) to the products we consume. And thus we intensify our addiction.

If the diabolical spirit, Hunger, lives inside your body and your mind, it's time to start the exorcism. The first step you must take is to accept that you need to change. It is obvious that your mind will always look for the quickest solution, for comfort. It happens to me: when the alarm goes off very early in the morning, I have the urge to switch it off; it's the easiest thing to do, "one extra hour of sleep". But I get out of bed because I am aware that I need to exercise —and I like it, of course. And I don't do it because I have more will power than you, of course not. But I decide to get out from under the covers and go and train. It's my choice. The same thing happens when it is time to eat: it is easier to order a pizza delivery— it gets there quickly, there's no need to cook— than to chop the broccoli, wash the other vegetables and then decide if they're going in the wok or simply into the salad bowl.

Every day, you and I make little decisions which can change our lives. Think about it properly: what will you do tomorrow? Will you repeat your dose of pancakes and sugar? Make the effort, make the decision from within, look for other breakfast options (or eating options in general). At the end of *The metabolic miracle* you will find some recipes which might help —yes, there are also desserts—. At first it won't be easy, but with the passing of the days you will begin to feel the change, the evil spirit will start to fade away and your life will be happier and more pleasant. It's as easy (and as hard) as saying: "Yes, I want to change". When you accept this change, you will enjoy each meal much more.

It's also very sad that, most of the time, we don't even look at the food we have on our plate. We don't even give thanks for being fortunate enough to have it. In restaurants I see a lot of robot-like children, who, while they press something on their tablet, open their mouth so that their mother or father can give them some fries with ketchup —full of sugar— or a piece of fried chicken with honey-flavored syrup —which isn't even honey—. The child doesn't know what they are eating. They don't care. But they learnt from their parents, who eat in the same manner. Everybody together, but separate, each one with their cellphone, taking apathetic bites of their hamburger, staring at the latest photo that their enemy posted on Instagram, or Kim Kardashian's cellulite in a paparazzi snap. Zombies created by the system.

You don't need a huge amount of will power to stop eating all day or set aside your cellphones when you get together at the table and be able to see, smell and understand what food you are going to put in your mouth and, above all, give thanks to life and the planet for this beautiful miracle you have before your eyes. If you are able to appreciate it, so too will your children; and they will teach the same thing to theirs. Let eating be something which brings us together, rather than separating us. May the force be with you!

"It's normal to be hungry all the time"

Yes, if we take into account that the dietary model has provoked this crazy and absurd eating anxiety. But the response should really be *no*. If your metabolism is in order, you shouldn't experience that insatiable appetite all the time. On a couple of occasions I have quoted the Harvard endocrinologist and pediatrician Doctor David Ludwig, who wrote a book on this subject which I recommend: *Always Hungry?*. In it, he explains a large part of what we have discussed here and analyzes in detail the effect which insulin has on the body. Ludwig reiterates that, if the levels of this hormone and its friends are elevated, due to the dietary model we have in the West in the 21st century, we will always be hungry. And that stimulus will be much stronger than our will power.

That is evidence of the neurohormonal condition we have been talking about in this chapter. That's why, if you are hungry all day, that could be a sign, or an early —or late— warning that something is not working in your metabolism. If this has not been happening for too long, take the necessary tests to verify if one of the indicators we have been discussing is suspect. If this has been happening for a while and you have put on weight and your tests show high triglyceride levels, fatty liver or elevated insulin levels, what are you waiting for to change your routines? Go over the previous sections! I tend to say that if you are hungry, you will always have the same possibilities as a traveler waiting for a train. If you listen for it in the distance, you will know it is on time and will be able to board. If you realize that it is approaching and you aren't very near to the platform, maybe you will make it on time and maybe you won't. And if you can't even hear it any more, your train has left the station. Don't let that happen.

There are a lot of factors which provoke continuous hunger. I have noticed that some of my patients who suffer from anxiety, for example, end up transferring their emotional condition, their problem, to food. Sometimes, these signs of internal discomfort, of not accepting who we are, stop us from taking a break and having a moment of reflection and clarity, to help make good decisions. And this creates another vicious cycle. **When faced with anxiety, many receive that impulse that they "have to eat". And they will usually eat something sweet. Sugar, with its addictive charm, will further stimulate the anxious symptoms of that person and their belief that they are "anxious". Anxiety will once again tell them that they "have to eat" and... eating and eating will generate more anxiety.** If you think this is happening to you, pull over onto the side of the road. Check your habits.

I see to cases like this very frequently. It's true that anxiety symptoms in some patients have some entirely provable physiological and biochemical triggers, but many are down to our deep-rooted beliefs; and from there we can transfer certain emotions to our food.

If you have managed to responsibly choose what you are going to eat, how you are going to fill your dish and when you will do it, it is a sign that your hormones are under control. The act of nourishing yourself will be a celebration without distress. I am sure that you won't be hungry all the time even if, one day, out of your own free will, you have chosen to eat just twice —we will talk about this sort of decision and controlled fasting at the end of the book—.

"You have to give the body what it asks for"

One of the decisive moments for the recovery of my patients who have developed a food addiction —due to the causes I described in the previous section— is when I ask them to eat three times a day, and not six or seven, as they have been doing for years. A short time after starting their new routine, the vast majority of them say to me: "Doctor! I can't. At 4:00 in the afternoon, my body asks me for [fill with whatever comes to mind] and I have to give it". The body asks them for "*dulce de leche*", meat pies, chocolate cake, "*chorizo and arepa*" (corn bread), strawberry ice-cream... every foodstuff on the face of the earth. Well, now that I come to think of it, none of them has told me that their organism asks them for broccoli, cauliflower or radishes.

This is the first sign of your own withdrawal symptoms, which you will soon get over. Some of them tell me that they have bad breath at mid-morning. Why? Because, as they tend to eat at that time, their body, out of habit and due to a neurohormonal effect, makes them salivate involuntarily and plentifully; that saliva leads to the bad breath.

What we all need to understand is that eating is not something that we do "because the body asks for it...". Eating should be the result of a conscious choice about what information to give our body and when we are going to give it. **Obviously, we all feel hungry, but it is a physiological mechanism which comes and goes in waves. It has been proven that those cravings to smoke, gamble, snort coke, have a drink or eat last for about four or five minutes.** That's not me, the functional heretic, saying it. Pavlov described it when he presented his studies on conditioned responses. I challenge you to try it for yourself. When you feel the call of the evil devouring spirit who lives inside you telling you: "The body is asking me for a *pain au chocolat* and a double cappuccino with whipped cream", take a breath and do the test. Doesn't the craving reduce over the minutes? Could you live without that pain au chocolat in the middle of the afternoon? Without doubt. A few pages ago I spoke to you about making decisions, this one was undoubtedly a very good one.

If only you knew my mother! While writing this section, I have thought about her a lot. Her metabolism is the only one of its kind on our planet. Her body asks her for sweet gelatin because the sweet gelatin levels in her blood are low. Or it asks her for cheese bread because the cheese bread levels in her blood are at a historic low. I believe that in Mom's hematic parameters, as well as hemoglobin, there is a special, annexed table which shows the following measurements: guava jelly level 14.5 mg/mbafi (where "mbafi" is "my body asks for it"), ripe plantain level 12.4 mg/mbafi... The worst thing about it is that I grew up under this belief model.

You don't need to give your body what it supposedly asks for. That impulse is not real. If, for years, you have been eating every three hours, or whenever your organism theoretically demands it, it is because you have a hormonal and neurohormonal disorder. But you can control it, you can change it. When we were kids and we had a bite which was really itchy, our wise parents would tell us: "Don't scratch it, if you scratch it, it will itch more". But, despite the warning, we scratched and, indeed, the itch got worse. The same exact thing happens in this case.

Do you know what your body is asking for? For you to feed it right.

"It's a sin to leave food on your plate"

Regardless of whether we have Catholic beliefs or not, we should abandon the use of the word "sin" when we are talking about the food that nourishes us. You are not a bad person because you left a piece of fillet and broccoli on your plate. If you are totally full, it doesn't make sense forcing your appetite. However, since we were little, our parents told you and me that it was a "sin" not to leave the plate completely clean, and that "there are lots of children in the world dying of starvation...". That's why we felt so terrible when it happens.

I am in no way condoning wasting food, but I also know that the majority of people who leave something on their plate are victims of the eating anxiety which grips the 21st century, and that anxiety makes them serve themselves more than their body can handle. And if we add to that the fact that people eat in a hurry and, especially, a lot of junk food, then we see results such as the "pizza effect" or "popcorn effect". I'm sure it has happened to you. You are at lunch with friends and you start to eat slices of pizza at a frantic pace. You have devoured two; then it's four. Six and you're still not full! But by the eighth piece you suddenly feel like you're about to explode —the same thing happens with the massive tubs of popcorn you buy at the cinema—. Why does this happen so suddenly if you felt as though you could eat three more entire pizzas? Because, while you were eating at full throttle, your brain still hadn't received the "warning" that you were in the midst of a pizza devouring session. This process can take, more or less, twenty minutes, and is a reflex which arrives via two routes; via the distension of the stomach and via a hormonal signal (leptin, which we spoke about earlier). That's why you suddenly feel full and wonder: "What happened, when did I eat so much?". And you will no doubt leave food on your plate.

A good strategy to avoid this happening is to eat slowly, chew your food repeatedly, impose a minimum time of 15 or 20 minutes for breakfast, lunch or dinner, and if you realize that you are finishing beforehand, you will know that you are actually eating too fast. Why are you in such a rush? Because you have to get back to work? Because you don't even care what you're eating? The act of feeding yourself and enjoying your dish is a moment for you to be "present", mindful of what you are doing, for at least a few minutes every day. I assure you that, if you take a bit more time to eat, it will be hard for you to leave food on your plate, because you will serve yourself the correct portion size. This is a good habit which your children will copy. The real "sin" is that you don't reflect on what you eat.

"Breakfast is the most important meal of the day"

I don't know if, in the rest of Latin America or the Motherland (Spain), the belief which is so rooted in my country, Colombia, exists, that you should breakfast like a king (i.e. eating plenty), lunch like a prince (again, eat a fair amount) and dine like a pauper (basically nothing). And on top of this idea is the other deep-rooted one, which you can see in the title of this section. Our grandparents and parents fostered that notion in our little infant brain. "Kid, you have to have a good —big— breakfast so that you have enough energy for the whole day". And, of course, you ended up vomiting on the school bus.

Lies! It isn't true. Picking up from what I have been telling you throughout the pages of this book, even if you haven't eaten all day —or for up to three days— you will have energy. Now, let me ask you, why? "Because we can make use of the energetic power of our second bodily turbine, whose fuel can be found in our body fat, doctor". Very good! You get a 10, a distinction.

I don't think that breakfast is the most important meal of the day. And, furthermore, we should know that eating immediately after getting up is not particularly recommendable. "Oh, no, doctor! Again with your ideas, now you're telling me I can't have breakfast?", you'll be thinking. It's not about that, calm down. But let's go over it again. Let's say it is 6:00 in the morning, you get out from under the covers, and your cortisol —the stress hormone— also wakes up clearheaded and in a good mood —it's your first load of the day—. The ideal situation, so that he can be relaxed, would be not to bother him for a couple of hours. That's why I made my previous suggestion: that time could be used to do some exercise on an empty stomach, for example.

But if you wake up at 6:00 in the morning and have breakfast at 6:30, you'll be giving your metabolism an extra job. When you eat, the insulin will be activated and it will interrupt the cortisol's awakening, making the whole metabolic process slower. And worse still if you have the breakfast of kings, with your four pancakes, two eggs, bacon, a XL coffee with sugar... Such a routine could ensure that you start to chronically put on weight. I know that some specialists claim that we should all eat immediately after waking up, because it is good for the thyroid. Although it isn't the star of *The metabolic miracle* —we would need a whole book just for that gland—, if your thyroid is affected by not eating, it is due to a chronic nutrient deficiency —I will touch on this topic a bit later.

So, in an ideal world, the recommended course of action would be to have breakfast two hours after waking up. And in that gap hopefully you can exercise. That way you will have a greater utilization of your cortisol and you will consume more of the glucose that you have stored in the liver and the body. I understand perfectly that modern life does not leave us with much spare time, that it can sometimes be impossible to have those two hours every day. However, give it a try. Is there any way you can rework your schedule?

While rats are nocturnal animals and eat at night, humans are day-dwellers and so our main meals should be consumed during the day. That does not mean that we need to feed ourselves first thing in the morning. If we go back in time and recall the history of our ancestors, who lived on this planet several thousand years ago, we will discover that the first thing they did when they woke up was go out in search of food. If they found any, they would be able to prepare something at around midday, eat in the afternoon and then go back out to do it again when it was dark and they would light a fire, shortly before going to sleep. If the male was going hunting in the morning, it would have been hard for the pre-historic Aunt Bertha to say: "Arlo, first you have to eat breakfast so that you have energy and don't get 'dizzy' when you are out hunting mammoths". Our ancestor's response would have been: "Auntie, what am I going to have for breakfast if there isn't anything? That's why I'm going hunting! Be right back".

That's how we have been for centuries. **I am sure that we didn't come to this earth in order to get up at 7:00 in the morning and immediately serve ourselves an enormous bowl of sugary breakfast cereal with lactose-free milk and a huge juice made from many oranges. The industry has encouraged us to be like that.** In the next section of the book we will talk in detail about what we could eat for breakfast and how.

Is breakfast the most important meal of the day? No. They are all important; in fact, in my opinion, lunch or dinner are more significant, provided you don't eat too late.

Part three

The metabolic
miracle

Chapter 9

What to eat

This is the first step in beginning to heal your metabolism. Perhaps yours has a slight disorder, or maybe you are severely affected. If you have paid attention to the chapters in this book, you will start to get a sense for it. It doesn't matter what state you are in, here you will find the initial solutions to improve it. The cure starts in your mouth, with the choices you make, with the information you give your organism. Using your mouth, you can correct hormonal problems, which are the cause of metabolic syndrome diseases, and thus take a step towards a better life.

It doesn't matter if you are a vegetarian, a vegan or a meat-eater, the way to regulate your metabolism is by maintaining a responsible, consistent and conscientious diet. This includes us all, no matter what our dietary preferences are, without creating segregations.

Don't eat that!

Let's begin. I recommend that you keep the following products, foods, preservatives, powders, additives and other "bad boys" far from your home and your life. By the way, don't keep a store of junk food for unexpected visits. What shouldn't you have at home?

1 › **No sugar.** Or honeys —least of all agave!— or natural or artificial sweeteners, no powdered fructose, no sweet chemicals which could be of use as an insecticide. "But doctor, how do I sweeten my coffee?". I repeat out loud: Coffee doesn't need sugar, especially if it is a good coffee! And remember the recommendations I gave you for that beverage.

2 › **Animal dairy**, especially from cows. Without drama, if the spirit living inside you one day asks for an ice-cream, look for a good one and get back to your good habits afterwards. No lactose-free, light or fat-free products. And don't forget that, if you get desperate and want a piece of cheese, it's better to choose a fatty, mature goat's or sheep's cheese. But, be strong, *bye bye* dairy for a good, long while (remember intestinal permeability).

3 › **Industrial cold cuts**, because they have too much sodium, a load of nitrites and a compound called monosodium glutamate, which raises uric acid levels. Only choose cold cuts which have undergone long curing and maturing processes. Read the labels! The majority of these contain sugars with identifiable names: sucrose, dextrose, malto-dextrin, syrups, among others.

4 › **Canned goods,** which also involve many chemical processes and include remains of heavy metals and too much monosodium glutamate.

5 › **Fruit juices**, whether they are shakes, smoothies or extracts, and that includes carrot and beet juices. I explained this in detail in this book. They are a *poison.*

6 › **Peanuts,** because they contain omega 6 —the excess of this fatty acid is affecting us all— and a toxin called aflato-xin, with a huge influence on liver cancer.

7 › **Processed food** with colorings and preservatives, and all products which boast of having "a smoked flavor" or use some weird word you can't even pronounce. Let's get back to natural products!

8 › **Alcohol.** Some drinks, like red wine, could have some form of short-term benefit; one or two occasional glasses can probably help with insulin resistance, but it has been proven that more than two glasses will have the opposite effect. Don't forget that alcohol is a carbohydrate and it behaves in a similar way to fructose. I like it, just like you, but if we want to heal our metabolism, the best thing to do is

avoid it. However, a glass of a good wine, a great single malt or an occasional —occasional!— beer don't represent a risk.

9 › Breakfast cereals and their cousins, granola, those which are packed with honeys and syrups. Please, remove them from your diet and that of your children.

10 › Bakery and patisserie products, and also those pastries we all like, made using any kind of flour. They all cause the same damage to the metabolism. It doesn't matter if they contain gluten or if the label certifies that they are gluten-free. At the end of the day, those who consume them regularly will end up being gluten-free but obese, with gluten-free fatty liver and a really cool gluten-free diabetes. The metabolic damage is the same. "And what about ketogenic baked goods, doctor?". They can be acceptable, but they disrupt the stomach acid and frequently cause acid reflux.

11 › Pasta. I should say that there are exceptions, but, *in general,* avoid it. In specific cases, which the functional doctor examines with their patients, pasta can be consumed. But if you are beginning the process of improving your metabolism, leave it out of your diet for a good while. Even gluten-free pasta.

12 › Pork, due to its high levels of histamine, which can produce an inflammatory response in the body, which raises cortisol levels and, why not, insulin levels too, especially in people who suffer from chronic allergies.

13 › Industrial sauces, ketchup, mayonnaise, mustard, soy sauce. Remember that you can make many of them at home, they taste better, and are sugar-free!

14 › Vegetable oils, canola, corn, sunflower or soybean, and products which contain them. Again: they are a very bad source of omega 6.

15 › "Hydrogenated" foods or margarines, that is, all those evil trans fats. Don't be taken in by the colorful warnings on the labels which say: "No cholesterol". Well of course they don't contain any: margarine comes from vegetables. It would be better and more honest for them to put a big warning which reads: "Spreadable trans fat".

16 › Aerosol foods (with very few exceptions). After all, you're looking for food, not a deodorant.

17 › Products with "cute", diminutive names, like many of those yogurts and chocolate milks for kids. That's not coming from me, my professor Mark Hyman said it, and he's right! The cuter the name, the more harmful its effect.

18 › The *Dirty Dozen*. These are the fruits and vegetables with a high chemical and pesticide content, and which are usually genetically modified. In the next section we will take a look at their good cousins, called the *Clean Fifteen*. For now, meet these twelve not-so-healthy actors, in order of their contamination levels: a) strawberries, b) spinach, c) nectarines, d) apples, e) grapes, f) peaches, g) cherries, h) pears, i) tomatoes, j) celery, k) potatoes, l) bell peppers. All foodstuffs with pesticides should be taken out of your diet.

Let me clarify: it doesn't mean that these vegetables are bad! If they are organic produce, if they come from small farms, they will bring joy to your body. If you can't find organic versions, try not to consume them in large quantities.

19 › Tert-Butylhydroquinone, TBHQ, a preservative derived from petroleum, better known as "lighter fluid". It is commonly used in margarines, breakfast cereals and some renowned chocolates which children love. Yummy! Chocolate with petroleum, how nutritional. It is also found in some types of peanuts and almonds.

20 › Products containing nitrites or nitrates, potassium bromate and parabens. There are two terrible compounds which are widely used as preservatives in children's breakfast cereals, BHT (Butylated hydroxytoluene) and BHA (beta hydroxy acid), and they are used in chewing gum!

21 › Foods with artificial flavoring. And be very careful with those which claim to use "natural flavorings". Some of them, like "natural" redcurrant or cranberry flavor —FDA approved— are derived from the anal glands of beavers, and sometimes these are put in breakfast cereals. At the end of the day, the industry doesn't lie, it is "natural", but not you, not I, not our children, want beaver butt for breakfast, right?

22 › The famous "caramel" coloring. The most well-known is the one used in the world's best-selling soft drinks brand. In fact, there is evidence that it is a producer and instigator of various forms of cancer. Obviously the United States Food and Drug Administration hasn't taken it into consideration. How many more deaths do there have to be for them to take it seriously? And you, how much "caramel coloring" do you drink per day?

23 › Perfect fruits and vegetables. I am talking, for example, about those round tomatoes which look as if they had been created by a set of compasses, with an impossible red color; they are so beautiful, so symmetrical, so perfect, that they are clearly genetically modified. The same applies to giant oranges, enormous shiny white onions and similar creations. Nothing that perfect is real. The consumer looks for aesthetic perfection, but doesn't think about the benefits of the product.

24 › Miracle shakes. Those which propose that the consumer replaces their breakfast with magic "powders" from a can. No chemical is a good substitute for real food. It has been proven that these products affect the bile duct —responsible for transporting bile between the liver and the gallbladder— and can provoke a lethal illness, called cholangitis. All of those shakes with names ending in *life*, which many well-known sportspeople promote, should be removed from your menu.

25 › Gym supplements. You already know their dangers. I have explained in great detail: be very careful with those "cocktails" of amino acids and sweet proteins, which look like the perfect shake when you add water. Be careful with all those chemicals contained in jars and tubs.

26 › Other compounds which shouldn't be in your diet are emulsifiers and some of the so-called gums. The former include carrageenan, which has lots of advocates because it is a derivative of seaweed, as if that makes it Poseidon's elixir or the secret mixture from which Mitch Buchannon —from *Baywatch*— receives nourishment. There are investigations which show that industrial carrageenan can cause colitis, digestive problems and can influence some forms of cancer. On the other hand, there are gums which are derivatives of trees and which can be good, and there are others which today are the most well-known way to hide the name *gluten*.

27 › **The plastic containers** we buy to store our food or which we use to take it to the office, are largely rich in derivatives like bisphenol A (BPA). It is also present in the plastic bottles which contain the water we buy or drink. What we don't know is that those bottles can spend months on a shelf and over time release their BPA into the liquid. This component —which is also found in the chemical paper used for receipts— has the capability to generate an excess of insulin and, therefore, a resistance to it. If we add this factor to a poor diet, sedentary lifestyle and bad habits, well, we're putting our health at risk. There are other plastic derivatives called phthalates —phthalic acid esters—, which are everywhere in your home: in PVC, in the paint on your walls, in the plastic curtains in the bathroom and in many of our younger children's toys, which they tend to put in their mouth! We especially need to protect them from phthalates, chemicals which you, Aunt Bertha and I, even though we might not want them, already have in our body. They can mainly affect the reproductive system and brain.

28 › **Imported meats** from countries with large, industrial production practices because, in general, the cows that the meat comes from have been fed on genetically modified grains, they have been given antibiotics to alter their gut

flora, which has provoked inflammation and insulin resistance and thus obesity —the fatter the specimens, the greater their value— and, what's more, they have been injected with hormones which create a race of suspect "bodybuilding" cows. You will eat all of these alterations that the animal has. If you live in one of these large nations, like for example the United States, ensure that the meat you are going to consume comes from grass-fed livestock. If you live in Latin America, you should have no problem finding it, almost all the local livestock is fed in this way.

29 › And what about salt? Good question! Many people want to remove it from their diet, but avoiding it is a mistake. I wanted to close this section on "What not to eat" with salt, because many people think that it is harmful. But no, if you look at the history of humanity, you will see that it has always been important. In fact, the word "salary" makes reference to the value in salt that somebody's work had.

Salt is totally necessary for the body. Today, we basically consume it in its sodium chloride form (NaCl) and we think that is the only one that exists. Oh yeah, and another really popular kind, created by marketing geniuses, is light salt, which has a higher potassium content. You already know what you can do with this type of product: not buy it! Ignore them and, if you have them, say goodbye to them.

Why, if sugar kills millions of people, do we keep extending its realm? Why, on the other hand, do we declare war on salt? For valid reasons: the excess of sodium in your body will favor the stagnation of liquid in your organism: you will have excess water in your tissues and blood vessels, which could lead to arterial hypertension and lead to other complications. However, the deficiency of salt is also linked to many diseases and cardiovascular conditions.

Don't ever forget that sodium plays a crucial role in your body, so much so that if the levels of this macromineral drop too much, you will die very quickly. If your levels of sodium and potassium are low, you will always be at risk.

I think I have cleared up one of your doubts: Do I have to include salt in my diet? Yes. But how do I create a balance of sodium and potassium in my body if conventional salt is not that "versatile"? One of the solutions is to consume foods which contain a good amount of one or the other, products high in sodium, like olives and nuts, and high in potassium, like spinach, broccoli, avocadoes, papaya and bananas, among others. Here's a side note. Yes, I said "spinach", and you must be shocked: "But doctor, you just told me that Popeye's vegetable of choice makes up part of the *Dirty Dozen*! And that I shouldn't consume it". Relax. I never told you that. I suggested that you look for a place where you can buy organic spinach. Spinach is very good! Let's move on.

If you want to enjoy the taste of salt, danger-free, the best thing for your palate and your body would be to buy a multi-mineral salt, such as Himalayan salt, which will give you that salty touch, but through the many minerals which it is made up of, and which are present in small concentrations.

However, you must be skeptical of my words because, for decades, Aunt Bertha has assured you that "any human being in their right mind should quit salt so as not to suffer from high blood pressure". Forget that advice. I think it is a mistake. You should include salt in your diet! But let me propose something: how about you cook your dishes without it and add it once they are served? I do it, it works for me and I do not sacrifice the taste of the dish I am going to eat. If you add it like this, it will be very close to the surface of the food on your dish and your tongue will quickly detect the salty flavor, so you will only have to add a little bit. If you add it while you are cooking, the salt will mix in with the other flavors but the sodium content will be absorbed into the dish.

In short: use salt with care and in moderation, do not remove it from your diet. Buy Himalayan salt or unprocessed sea salt, which is very good. And always avoid the added salt in industrial foodstuffs. If you want to expand your knowledge of this great source of sodium, I recommend reading *The Salt Fix* (2017), by Doctor James DiNicolantonio.

When my editors and I went over this chapter one last time, we thought that this is right about the point where you will want to: a) close the book, b) burn this book!, c) faced with the desperation of not finding anything good to eat, eat the pages of this chapter —with a bit of Himalayan salt. In fact, I think that could be a very interesting niche, edible books, high in good carbohydrates, high in healthy fats and proteins— and sugar-and gluten-free! Unfortunately, the idea didn't go down too well with the executives at the publishing house. So. Don't close this book, don't burn it and don't eat it. I know this list seems distressing. I know that, right now, you must be angrily saying: "This Jaramillo guy has messed up my existence! Now I won't be able to have a social life! And what am I going to give my kids to eat? I'm off to buy some pork scratchings with a soft drink, topped off with three desserts, and I'll forget this whole thing!". Or how about you have a little patience, keep reading and let us talk about what we should eat? With a little bit of calm, some discipline and will power, and lots of awareness, you are going to take an important step for your life. It will be easy, and appetizing, too.

Please, eat this

Don't expect impositions from my part. I am not going to give you a strict menu telling you what to eat each day. Nor am I going to suggest you go to restaurants with a little "scale" to weigh the servings of each macronutrient (carbohydrates, fats and proteins) or that you download the latest calorie counting apps —a useless exercise—. I am going to ask you to do something which may sound contradictory: relax! "But doctor, how am I supposed to relax if, throughout this book, you've been telling me to drop bread, milk, juice and even pasta? There's nothing left for me to eat!", you might argue. And with good reason.

Let's go step by step. Here I am going to give you some recommendations which will help you, and in the next chapter I will explain how you can combine them, mix them, and transform them so that, in the midst of all this information and your new habits, you don't lose your mind when you are invited to the newest *trattoria*, recommended by food critics, and are lost without your script. Let's start with the macronutrients which should be the stars of your culinary movie: good carbohydrates.

Lots of vegetables!

They should never be absent from your dish. "But doctor, lettuce and I don't have any chemistry!", you will explain in distress. There is life beyond this green leaf, although I think it's fantastic. Remember that there isn't just *one* lettuce, there is an enormous variety. And with a great vinaigrette and the right partners, it is food from the big leagues. But the world of vegetables is very extensive. Don't limit yourself. Let your guard down. I suggest that you include fibrous green vegetables in your diet, such as kale, spinach and, yes, lettuce! But remember to combine them with vegetables of various colors; be your salad's graphic designer, painter, or artist, use the full Pantone palette and make sure there is green (like the ones I mentioned), red (tomatoes, bell peppers, radishes, among others), yellow (zucchini, bell peppers and similar products), white (cauliflower, palm hearts, garlic, onions, asparagus, mushrooms, to name a few) and purple (beets, red cabbages, eggplant, various lettuces). And you can rotate them each day. Include a lot of vegetables in your meals.

"Doctor, can I eat potatoes? And what about plantain and rice?", my patients frequently ask me when we begin their metabolic recovery. And I tend to respond: all in good time. At the start of the diet I prefer to set them aside, but then we will begin to re-incorporate them —it depends on the progress of each person—. Over time, your plate can include cereals (rice, quinoa, couscous, among others) and starches (potatoes, yucca, plantains, sweet potatoes), but don't forget that both groups are essentially fiber and glucose. However, at the start of the process, it is best to exclude them, remember that we are correcting your metabolism. While we ensure that your blood indicators and body fat percentage are at correct levels, stay true to your starter vegetables.

Fruit, of course

But the best way to include it in your diet is at breakfast time. I don't recommend it at dinner time —at night— and do not include it between meals. How many servings of fruit should you consume a day? According to what the World Health Organization published in August, 2018, "at least 400 grams (or, five servings) of fruit" a day. This recommendation seems excessive to me. I make this assertion based on the work I have done, alongside my patients, to achieve the correction of their metabolism. The results we have obtained allow me to recommend that, if you do not have metabolic problems, you could eat up to two daily servings of fruit —*with* your meals—; and if some form of metabolic disorder has been detected, one serving should be enough, until your organism gets back to normal.

"And what kind of fruit, doctor?". Preferably those with a low glycemic load and low glycemic index. The latter, as I have already explained, refers to the available glucose capacity that a person has in their blood after having eaten a food —in this case fruit— and how much the levels of said glucose rise. The glycemic load is the amount of "sugar" per centimeter contained in a foodstuff, and will be high or low depending on whether its consumption produces an increase in the blood sugar levels over a long period or short period. Above all, here we are looking at the intensity of the insulin response to the food being received.

To answer more directly, include those which have more fiber in your diet, and especially those with lower glycemic indices and loads, like strawberries (organic), raspberries, blackberries, cranberries, grapefruits, kiwis, pineapples, oranges, lemons, limes, cape gooseberries, coconuts, green apples, green or slightly ripe mangoes, among others.

A lot of fruits don't include the mentioned properties and are still good. Take, for example, the watermelon. It has very little fiber and a high glycemic index (70); in fact, many nutritionists condemn it because of that. But, on the other hand, it has a low glycemic load, which means that its concentration of fructose per centimeter is very low. Watermelon is, basically, water. Do you see? High index, but *low* load. A point in favor of watermelons. The world isn't perfect. Neither are fruits. However, I reiterate, the best option would be a fruit which has both of the previous at "low" levels, and better still a good fiber contribution.

I haven't forgotten: in the last section I told you about the *Dirty Dozen* —the twelve fruits and vegetables with the most pesticides— and I promised to give you the list of the *Clean Fifteen*, which, by contrast, are those with the least traces of pesticides. Here they are: 1) avocadoes, 2) sweetcorn —only consume it if it is organic so as not to eat a genetically modified mutant—, 3) pineapples, 4) cabbage, 5) onions, 6) peas, 7) papaya, 8) asparagus, 9) mangoes, 10) eggplants, 11) cantaloupes, 12) kiwis, 13) grapefruits, 14) cauliflower and 15) broccoli.

Healthy fats

I have told you this in detail in many parts of this book. Healthy fats are beneficial for your body and should be a permanent fixture in your diet. Throughout the history of humanity, our forefathers consumed them tirelessly. Where to find these good fats? In olive, coconut, avocado or sesame oils (remember: no vegetable oils like canola or sunflower); in whole coconuts, avocadoes, olives; in nuts like almonds, cashews, macadamias, pecans, walnuts (don't buy those which have been toasted in vegetable oil!); in seeds like chia, sunflower, linseed, sesame, hemp; in fish such as salmon, in eggs, cacao and ghee (clarified butter). Include these in your diet every day; I will give you more instructions in a few pages' time.

Animal proteins

If you are going to eat red meat, it's best that it comes from grass-fed livestock, as is the case in our region. Avoid the famous American Angus meats. There are other very good sources of animal protein which are not so common, such as lamb, duck and turkey, which also offer a first-class complement, healthy fats! If you are going to eat chicken, make sure it is organic, from the countryside, that it hasn't been fattened up using antibiotics or genetically modified corn, and that it doesn't have an excess of sodium. It's not an impossible task, ask, check, no doubt there is a place near your neighborhood where you can find it, but maybe you don't know about it because you always buy it at the supermarket.

It is often believed that the healthiest protein option is fish, but it is the most contaminated species of all; it is a victim of human "progress". Their marine or river habitats are contaminated with mercury, arsenic, industrial waste, fecal matter, plastic and dozens of toxins that have become their food because of us. I suggested this many pages ago, when we talked about omegas: try to consume the smallest fish on the food chain —like sardines, for example— because they will always be the least contaminated. Here we can really say that their size is directly proportional to their toxicity. Avoid swordfish —it isn't very common in our countries, but there are those who may succumb to the charms of "exotic" food— and only consume fresh tuna, once a month —never canned—. Some gym and weights enthusiasts start to eat an absurd amount of this good fish with the aim of increasing and defining their muscle mass. They will probably achieve the desired result on the outside, but they will be making themselves sick on the inside. Is it worth it? One might think that farmed fish do not have the aforementioned problems, but that depends on their food source; if they are fed with grains, rejected!

"And is it true, doctor, that eating liver is bad?". I'm glad you asked that. This offal contains many nutrients that the body needs; however, it has a very bad reputation due to a misunderstanding. It is true that it is the organ which carries out the majority of the organism's detoxification, but what is not explained is that the majority of the toxins accumulate in the fat and not the liver. If you want to eat it, do it —but make sure it comes from a good source—.

I am not going to mention dairy proteins because, as I explained in the chapter dedicated to milk, if we weigh up the benefits and the damage that they bring to your body, the latter will win. The same applies for pork.

Eggs

Eggs are a great source of animal protein, of course, but I did not want to include them in the previous section because they have their distinctive features. They have many benefits, as well as many critics. What's more, eggs also offer up a good amount of healthy fats; they are a "two for one" deal. However, they provoke disagreements: even today, there is no consensus among nutrition specialists about how many eggs we can eat a day. It isn't easy to set a guideline because many people are allergic or show signs of sensitivity to eggs —like my wife, some time ago—. And, furthermore, this foodstuff receives a lot of bad press. Aunt Bertha, for example, says that "eggs raise your cholesterol", a false statement which I ask you to forget. In general, if your metabolism is fine, if you know that you are not allergic or sensitive to them, you can eat two to three eggs a day, and not necessarily for breakfast. This routine will not raise your cholesterol or cause a heart attack, I assure you.

Eggs also contain multiple essential vitamins for the development and regeneration of tissues. They complement the nervous system and contribute to the upkeep of involuntary functions such as sleep, relaxation, digestion, hormone production and many others, through a powerful nutrient called choline, which it contains plenty of. It is the precursor molecule for a compound which is very important to our body, acetylcholine, a neurotransmitter of vital importance.

We could dedicate dozens of pages to eggs, but that would take us on an unnecessary thematic detour. I'll be satisfied if you understand that they are a superfood. They have so many advantages that a living being can be born from them! When can your children include them in their diet? After their first year, without any problem. What kind of eggs to buy? Organic. Look, it is not important if they come from chickens who run wild and free or who dance ballet, the main point is that you ensure they have been produced by well-fed, well-looked after country hens. If you happen to find ones which are organic and also omega 3 enriched —which come from chickens who had seaweed as a dietary su- pplement—, fantastic! But they are not easy to find in Latin Ame- rican countries. If they are organic you can rest easy, you will have a good source of protein and fat for you and your family. And eggs are really versatile! They can be cooked in many different ways.

Plant proteins

Before continuing, I think it is appropriate for me to make this clarification: there is no natural foodstuff which is just protein or just carbohydrates; almost all of them have, in varying degrees, a number of macronutrients in their structure. As I explained seve- ral chapters ago, meat is not just protein, it is also made up of fats, fiber and water. The same applies to the vegetables you will find in this section. They are still carbohydrates, but they have a high pro- tein content. It is important that this is clear so that you don't get wrapped up in misunderstandings. Of which there are many. At lunches with work colleagues who decide to go to a "healthy" res- taurant, it is common to hear phrases like "quinoa is a superpro- tein". No. Above all, quinoa is a carbohydrate, it is a grain which contains a good amount of protein, ok? That is different.

I tell you this because, if you start to consume it in excess thin- king solely about its protein content, you are going to generate a metabolic disorder in your body because it is, above all, a carb, which will end up altering your insulin levels. Don't fall into the trap. Understand what you are eating and why.

The most commonly used plant proteins are pulses, like beans, chickpeas and lentils; mushrooms; edamame and tofu, both of which come from soybean —which should be certified and non-genetically modified; broccoli and nuts, the ones we talked about in the section on fats: almonds, macadamias, cashews and their cousins—.

Although grains are a good source of protein and are very tasty, patients with autoimmune diseases worry about consuming them because they contain lectins, which can produce intestinal damage —just like gluten, which is a lectin— and worsen their condition. However, if you suffer from one of these conditions and want to eat grains, you can as long as you follow this simple method: soak them for several hours in water with lemon and apple cider vinegar, wash them, and then also cook them in water with lemon and cider vinegar. Goodbye lectins! And *bon appetit.*

I almost forgot: in general, sesame paste, known as tahini —a culinary jewel from the Arabs and the Turks— is another food which you can include in your diet, alongside pure nut butters —with no added vegetable oils— and chickpea hummus, or eggplant, cauliflower and avocado dips. See? There are a lot of options. You don't just have to eat lettuce —in any case, in a few weeks, you and green or red lettuce will be the best of friends—.

Spices

These have tremendous powers and qualities. For thousands of years they have been used in different cultures to improve the taste of food, but also for healing the body. One of these is turmeric, used for centuries in traditional Chinese medicine. Numerous studies on its effectiveness and purpose show that it is the most powerful anti-inflammatory in existence. Turmeric has an influence on the same spots in our body where the industry's most well-known commercial anti-inflammatories, such as ibuprofen and corticosteroids act. You could say that, by consuming this spice, you are regulating the same areas that said medicines affect. In order to activate the turmeric and ensure it is absorbed better, I recommend you lightly toast it in a dry frying pan with black pepper. That way, you will also add the anti-inflammatory properties of the latter.

I wanted to focus on turmeric because it is not that popular in our region —we should use it more—, but there are a lot of other spices waiting for you to include them in your diet, among those cloves, cinnamon —to control the production of and resistance to insulin—, ginger —another anti-inflammatory—, thyme, oregano, bay leaves and cilantro —they have antimicrobial properties and help to remove the excess of gut flora—. There are a lot of spices and chilies, such as cayenne pepper, which are also anti-inflammatories.

One of the rock stars of the spice family is garlic, which is present in almost all the homes in the world and gives a wonderful kick to meals. Garlic joins the list of anti-inflammatories —thanks to its sulfur molecules called trisulfites—, also contains antimicrobial properties —antiviral and antiparasitics— and it can be consumed by everyone, but not at every moment in life. Why? If you have a good memory you will remember. I told you in the first part of the book: garlic is rich in fructans and these can raise the uric acid levels. Some people are victims of this; let's say they have a delicious dinner at night, with dishes full of garlic, but when they wake up the next morning they feel like they have put on ten kilos —I'm exaggerating, but that's the idea—. "What happened?", they wonder. "No doubt it was the potatoes". But no. "Or the roast beef". Not that either. It was Mr. Garlic's fault, but he never gets the blame. And this happens because these people have a metabolic problem: this spice's fructans cause a crisis and the organism retains a lot of liquid. What is the reason? Chronic inflammation. All of the body's inflammatory routes lead to water retention! Always. In short, be careful with garlic.

"And what about onions, doctor? You said something about them and fructans". It's true. They produce the same problem as the rock star of the spice world, except they do not have any anti-inflammatory properties. That doesn't mean that you can't eat them. There are other foods which also raise uric acid levels, I won't name them here, because they act differently in each individual; I analyze them in my consultations, with every patient and with their most recent uric acid tests; I tend to work to values which are very different to those traditionally accepted by the majority of laboratories, which can be very permissive.

Liquids

Let's start with an undeniable scientific fact: all human beings are basically water, 60 % of our organism is water, our cells are full of water. And we need to drink it, but it has to be good and healthy.

What runs through the pipes and comes out of the taps in each country is different and has different properties. It is drinkable, sure, but that does not mean it is the most suitable for our body. So, what should we drink? I would recommend filtered water; there are various brands offering good filters, choose the one you want. The investment will be worth it and allow you to steer clear of plastic bottled water, with its BPA, which we mentioned earlier. If the liquid is bottled in glass, there is no risk of contamination.

Some years ago, lots of people started to look for alkaline drinks or to drink water with bicarbonate of soda and lemon, on an empty stomach, in order to alkalize their bodies. This has been one of the 21st century's trends. And does it help? Well at least it doesn't intoxicate you, but its benefits are, above all, an urban legend. Why are you looking for this alkalinity? "Because I have gastritis, doctor, like everybody else", you may explain. I get it, what you're saying is logical, but for the hundredth time, our body doesn't work like that. The stomach in its natural state is acidic and, although it sounds contradictory, we should keep it that way.

I had chronic gastritis because, like most earthlings, in my childhood I ate breakfast cereals, drank soft drinks which make Life Taste Good and had some shocking eating habits. Over the years, and with the acquired knowledge, I was able to control the gastritis —without the help of pills or magical elixirs—. I understood this: to escape from the grips of gastritis, you have to preserve the stomach's physiology, its acidity, not try to eradicate it. Here is my favorite "potion" for keeping the stomach in an ideal condition: water, lemon and/or apple cider vinegar. I drink it all day, even as I am writing these lines. It's no myth. It's no urban legend. It's a very useful liquid, which has added results, such as controlling insulin, uric acid and cortisol. And it is also a magnificent indicator of how your stomach is doing. If you can't take this drink, if it doesn't go down too well, if it causes you a lot of "acidity", that is a sign that you need to start a process of healing, because anybody should be able to handle it without any problems.

Do it. Water, a squeeze of lemon, a splash of apple cider vinegar —make sure it's organic and that the label says "with The Mother", that's the good stuff—. If your stomach is fine, you will have good nutrient absorption and not be inflamed. But after sharing so many pages with you, I've started getting to know you, so I should warn you that this "potion" will do you no good if you keep eating badly and at all hours, if you also drink a lot of alcohol, don't sleep the required amount of hours and don't try to cut down that 16-hour work day which you consider so normal and productive.

We should all drink between a liter and a half and two liters of water or fluids a day, but keep in mind that many of the foods that you eat are rich in fluids; I'm talking about lettuce —your best friend— or watermelon, to give but two examples. That contribution helps. What else can I drink? Tea (not bottled); there are good teas everywhere these days, go to your favorite store and speak to the manager and have them explain their properties; learn to prepare them: black tea, rooibos (red bush) tea, white tea, matcha tea —powdered green tea— and, best of all, at least for me, green tea, which you can drink at any time. But don't go over the top! What is the bad thing about tea? The caffeine. Please, be very aware of that, we will soon talk about it. And don't forget to drink fruit and vegetable infusions which are really good; this is another world for you to discover, mix and enjoy.

If you started reading this book back to front and are wondering why I have not recommended drinking fruit juices or smoothies, go to the chapter on fructose and you will understand. For now, I have a couple more liquid guests, who I will talk about in the next two sections. Let's begin with plant-based milk and then move on to the misunderstood dark drink.

Plant-based milks

They have gained popularity around the world and it is fairly clear to see. Today, 70 % of the world population is lactose intolerant —all of the planet's inhabitants should be but we have already discussed that in the chapter on dairy— and people have not given up on the search for a substitute to calm their milk cravings. Yes, it is true that a large handful of the people looking for these white liquids do so because they understand that they can be better for their organism. We call them "milks", but in reality they are vegetable drinks made from almonds, coconuts and cashews, among others —I don't include soymilk here, which I mistrust, due to all the genetic transformations this seed has undergone—. However, to be precise, technically we can call them "milks" because they undergo lactic fermentation and this process is not unique to animal dairy. I'll just leave that clarification there for the purists and specialists from the world of cow's milk.

I always recommend that my patients learn to make them at home; it isn't very complicated. "Oh no, doctor, don't be such a hippie, I don't have the time or a machete at home to chop coconuts!", you will desperately be shouting right about now. Hopefully you will try it out. But, if you definitely don't have the time, look for them in places which can guarantee their preparation method. At the supermarket I see more and more people buying almond milk; I dare say that they are doing it because a friend recommended it to them. They go to the "healthy" food aisle and take the first one they see. And they don't read the label! And they end up buying a mass-produced drink with a pitiful almond content. Perhaps, if they had stopped to check the information on the carton, they would realize that that "milk" contains less than 8 % almonds and that the remaining content is made up of chemicals, colorings and thickeners.

Get out your calorie-counting calculator. Have you got it? Good, let's do some mathematical calculations. So you bought a carton of almond milk which says that each glass contains 30 CAL. Perfect. A single almond has seven CAL. So that glass contains 4.28 almonds. If you take 4.28 almonds and blend them, you will never get a liquid as thick as the one which comes out of the carton. What is the secret? That the rest of the glass is made up of thickeners and emulsifiers, exactly what you shouldn't consume, but go ahead and drink your little glass of chemicals. To top it all off, some of these milks contain sugar, and others are even worse: they are mixed with soybean, canola or sunflower oil —highly inflammatory, bad sources of omega 6. Look for a good almond milk or coconut milk— this is my favorite, I know it well (remember that I am allergic to almonds) —or cashew milk—. Don't drink them as a punishment, don't drink them hoping that they will taste like cow's milk. My dear reader-calf, I said it from the beginning: these are not "animal milks". They could even be better than that.

Coffee

I am lucky enough to live and have been born in a country which has a considerable variety of coffees. It's a cliché, yes, but it's true. I have verified it. When I have lived far away, I have always missed Colombian coffee. Play the national anthem! But this drink, so popular all over the world, is one of the great misunderstood beverages. It's the same as with garlic, *everyone* can drink coffee, but *not all* the time and with the same frequency and in the same way. This is a great liquid, it has antioxidants which help fight chronic inflammation and the damage caused by free radicals. What's more, it contains good fats, but the component which makes it unique is, at the same time, its worst enemy: caffeine. Which is also contained in the teas we spoke about not too long ago, remember?

Caffeine stimulates adrenaline, a hormone and neurotransmitter which works with the nervous system and which is responsible for preparing the body to activate the state of "fight or flight". In this state of alarm, the heart beat and blood pressure rise, the pupils dilate —because a much clearer field of vision is required in order to escape—, all of the circulation is sent to the extremities and the blood flow to the organs is cut.

In the process of stimulating adrenaline, a signal is sent to the adrenal glands to produce cortisol, the stress hormone. And careful with this: if you have an imbalance in the hormonal axis which goes from your brain to the adrenal glands, each time you drink coffee you will produce more adrenaline, which will then stimulate the creation of cortisol, and in the midst of all this chaos more insulin will be produced, and if this gets together with uric acid, it's every man for himself! And it all started because of a small stimulus generated by a drink which, on the whole, should be beneficial for your body.

Coffee is delicious, but it is not the most suitable fluid for those who know they have problems with their cortisol; for everybody else, it is. Under normal circumstances, we can all drink between one or two cups a day —mainly in the morning and up to midday at the latest—. But, getting back to what I have repeated incessantly throughout the book; look for a good product, buy a good coffee, ideally organic, from high in the mountains, better yet if you can get the whole bean, if it wasn't toasted too long ago, and if you can grind it at home —the price of electric coffee grinders has lowered, they are small, convenient and quick—. It will be a pleasure for your body, and better still if it's Colombian, of course.

"Doctor, why is it better to drink it in the morning?". Because that is when your organism has the most cortisol. In that state, if your body experiences an adrenaline spike from the coffee, you will be fine. If you drink it at night, for example, it can induce an adrenaline and cortisol spike at a time when they should be decreasing and getting ready for bed. "So, doctor, what about my afternoon coffee?". Drink a *good* decaffeinated coffee, every day they are making better ones, but bear in mind that there are two ways to decaffeinate: 1) by chemical extraction and 2) by rinsing. Hardly anyone is told this, so be sure to ask the barista at the place you tend to buy your coffee. Ideally you want a coffee which has been decaffeinated by rinsing.

Oh, and I almost forgot Aunt Bertha, who was very interested in this chapter. She stopped drinking coffee because, according to her own theory, it is synonymous with gastritis. If you feel the same way as she does when you drink a cup of coffee, then no doubt your stomach acidity is off and you have irritated mucous membrane. Let me explain. Just as you have your sympathetic nervous system, which controls the states of fight or flight in your body, you also have its opposite, the parasympathetic nervous system, which manages sleep, relaxation, digestion, breathing, states of calm and peace, controls the secretion of hormones and is responsible for making the glands carry out all their processes. What's more, it manages the stomach's acid production. This organ needs to preserve its acidity, but when you drink coffee, which contains caffeine and stimulates the adrenaline, well, you are giving the sympathetic system an alarm signal, which is why the production of acid in the stomach is stopped and the mucous becomes irritated. However, coffee is not guilty for gastritis.

Vinegars and fermented foods

Other products you can incorporate into your diet are healthy condiments such as mustard —not the one which comes in suspicious tubs in the supermarket—, healthy oils such as olive, avocado and coconut oil, for example; vinegars such as balsamic and apple cider "with The Mother" (the important thing is that they are not reduced with sugar); homemade mayonnaise, prepared using good fats and eggs; fermented foods such as sauerkraut —made with cabbage—, kimchi —a Korean creation— and kombucha —a drink made from fermented tea—. This last one on the list is recommended in small quantities (half a cup a day), because, as with any fermented foodstuff, if it is consumed in excess it can raise the uric acid levels. I see many people choosing to drink it because it is cool (it's fashionable) and they drink it uncontrollably. You should investigate what you are drinking better.

Chapter 10

How to eat what you should eat

You now know what to keep out of your life and off your dish. You also know what to include in your three daily meals. Here I am going to explain how you can find a good balance of these foods and how you can "calculate", intuitively and without electronic devices, the serving size of each of the valuable macronutrients which you will give your body every time you sit down at the table, alone, with friends or with family.

The basis of every dish should be carbohydrates

Mainly vegetables. As I told you in the last chapter, and at the risk of sounding repetitive, in order to start correcting your metabolism without pills that leave stains on your underwear, without telesales products, without miracle recipes or jungle products prepared by a shaman, you have to start by changing your eating habits and understanding that your first great allies are vegetables. That is the starting point. But, as we begin generating the necessary corrections to your organism, you need to keep grains and starches off your plate for a while, including rice, quinoa, potatoes, yucca, plantains, sweet potatoes, squash, beets and corn. Maybe you could, every once in a while, eat half an arepa (Colombian corn bread) for breakfast. But only for breakfast; don't include it in your dinner. "How many centuries will this torture last, doctor?". Don't be so dramatic. The time that this process takes will depend on how committed you are to your new habits. When your blood levels, your weight and your body fat percentage return to normal levels, you will have reached the time when you can rediscover grains and starches. Don't rush it.

Ready for the first step? **I know that you are used to exact measurements, the precise numbers provided to you by your cellphone or smartwatch, which register the number of steps you take, your heart rate, how many kilometers you covered, how many calories you burned. Now I want to request that you set your devices aside and, at a glance, simply with the help of your sight and common sense —which is an app that we rarely use—, calculate that your dish always contains 75 % vegetables.** Remember that proportion: three quarters of your meals should be vegetable origin carbohydrates. Using these, your organism will be able to produce all the glucose that it wants, and even proteins, because vegetables are full of amino acids.

"No, doctor, what do you mean? Could you be a bit more precise?". OK. Easy, make a big salad. "And what do I put in it?". Start with green fibrous vegetables —include your best friends, lettuce (green, leaf, romaine, red, iceberg), kale, spinach, arugula (its bitter touch is delicious)— and create your own design on top of this green palette, like I told you in the previous chapter: include various colors, flavors, raw or cooked vegetables, and make a nice dressing, with extra virgin olive oil, apple cider vinegar —organic and with The Mother— or balsamic vinegar and a bit of Himalaya salt. If you want, add chia seeds or some nuts. The most beautiful thing about "designing" your salad is that you have endless possibilities. Or, alternatively, get out your wok or deep pan and prepare some nice sautéed vegetables. As you can see, there are numerous options. But please, don't use the microwave oven to heat or cook your vegetables; in fact, don't use the microwave at all, you don't need that radiation in your food. Are there parents in the audience? One recipe which children tend to love is zucchini pasta. I recommend it. To sum up, if you can make this the basis of your diet —and probably that of your family too—, you will be giving your body an enormous offering of vitamins, minerals and antioxidants.

Ensure you eat the appropriate amount of protein for you

If you have a good memory, you will remember that we spoke about this issue in the second part of *The metabolic miracle*. Let me get back to that initial approach. This book is written for everyone and all their dietary choices, but in order to explain the protein contribution of your diet, I will use animal meat, which makes up the protein contribution of the majority of humans on the planet. And this time I will explain it in a more detailed manner.

1 › Approximately 25 % of the weight of white meat and around 30 % of the weight of red meat is effective protein.

2 › That is to say that, if you are going to consume 100 grams of white meat or seafood, more or less 25 grams of that will be effective protein. If we're talking about red meat, it will

be 30 grams. These are not absolute, exact, perfect figures but they will make it easier for you to make your protein calculation.

3 › If you don't do much physical activity —you get up, go to work, exercise from time to time and don't have any interest in being Mr. Muscle—, you should consume between 0.8 and 1 gram of protein for every kilo that you weigh.

4 › If you are a woman and are 1.60 meters tall, your ideal weight should be —more or less— 55 kilos, so you should consume 55 grams of protein.

5 › Let me give you an example of this consumption: you eat an egg in the morning (7 grams of effective protein), a 100 gram serving of salmon at lunch (25 grams of effective protein) and a 100 gram serving of chicken for dinner (25 grams of effective protein), to make a total of 57 grams of effective protein that day. It doesn't matter if the figure isn't exactly the same as your weight, the important thing is getting close.

6 › Now let me ask you: if you are 1.60 meters tall but weight 90 kilograms, how much protein should you consume? Right now I hope you will say to me: "Well, the very same 55 grams, doctor, because the protein contribution is calculated according to the ideal weight, so 55 kilos". And right about now I am crying with joy. You are completely right.

7 › Never forget: the calculation of how much protein a person needs is always based on their ideal weight and not their current weight.

Now let's do the same exercise with a man who also carries out moderate levels of physical activity.

1 › Suppose you are 1.85 meters tall. Therefore, your ideal weight should be 80 kilos —more or less—. That means you need a protein intake of 80 grams.

2 › How do you do it? Let's say that you eat two eggs for breakfast, which represent 14 grams of effective protein. For lunch you satisfy yourself with 120 grams of beef, or 36 grams of effective protein. At dinner you eat 120 grams of duck, at a special celebratory meal, which gives you a contribution of 30 grams of effective protein. In total you consumed 80 grams of effective protein throughout the day, so that's perfect.

Yes, you have other doubts, one of which will be: "Doctor, how do I know how many grams the servings I am going to eat are?". Taking into account your weight, ask your butcher to cut the meat into pieces which allow you to achieve the desired protein intake. If we go back to the example of the man who is 1.85 meters tall and whose ideal weight should be 80 kilos, he should ask for pieces which weigh between 120 and 150 grams. "And what if I go to a restaurant? Should I take some scales?". No. If you go to a restaurant, relax and enjoy yourself; and use the "eyemeter", or visual measurements, along with your common sense app. "Doctor, I regularly and actively participate in physical training, should I eat more or less proteins?". I would recommend that you consume up to 1.5 grams of effective protein per kilo of body weight.

"Doc, what I want is to build lots of muscle mass with my training, is it true that I should eat a lot of protein to build muscle?". Good question. Some authors suggest that a person with your ambitions should eat up to 3 grams of protein per kilo. I do not share their assessment. Eating a whole load of proteins does not guarantee more muscle formation. Muscle grows and forms with appropriate training, focused on achieving that goal. Don't forget that an excess of protein will make your body produce more glucose and can also be a bad stimulus for your genes and perhaps end up causing cancer. "Oh, doctor, don't be so fatalistic, you're beginning to sound like Aunt Bertha". It isn't fatalism. It's prevention. If you don't believe me, I suggest you read *The China study*, by Doctor T. Colin Campbell.

Before moving on to the next section, remember that all of those magnificent proteins which we have spoken about must be joined on their plate by those wonderful vegetable carbohydrates and your bestie, lettuce. They are the perfect complements on your culinary palette. Here is a table so that you can calculate how many grams of protein certain foods provide.

MEAT	
Beef (170 grams)	54 grams
Turkey, breast (170 grams)	51.4 grams
Pork chop (170 grams)	49 grams
Turkey, dark meat (170 grams)	48.6 grams
Hamburger (170 grams)	48.6 grams
Chicken, dark meat (170 grams)	47.2 grams
Tuna (170 grams)	40.1 grams
Grilled steak (170 grams)	38.6 grams
Chicken, breast (170 grams)	37.8 grams
Ham (170 grams)	35.4 grams
Salmon (170 grams)	33.6 grams

DAIRY/EGGS	
Soy milk (177 milliliters)	6.7 grams
Eggs (1 large)	6.5 grams

MEAT SUBSTITUTES/GRAINS/ LEGUMES AND NUTS	
Veggie hamburger (170 grams)	51.4 grams
Tofu (170 grams)	13.8 grams
Almond butter (2 tablespoons)	7 grams
Lentils (1/2 cup)	9 grams
Split peas (1/2 cup)	8.1 grams
Beans (1/2 cup)	7.6 grams
Sesame seeds (28 grams)	7.5 grams
Black turtle beans (1/2 cup)	7.5 grams
Chickpeas (1/2 cup)	7.3 grams
Peas (1/2 cup)	4.1 grams

Healthy fats should never be missing from your three daily meals

Healthy fats are absolutely crucial and necessary for ensuring a good balance in each of your dishes. I recommend that my patients include between two and four types of healthy fat in each of their meals. How? Let me give you some tips; these are just examples.

1 › At breakfast, for example, prepare your eggs with coconut oil and, be bold, eat half an avocado —yes, for breakfast—. Right there you have three healthy fats: eggs, coconut and avocado. You can also mix coconut or almond milk with chia seeds to make a pudding, which you can accompany with nuts and cinnamon.

2 › For lunch, eat a big salad with olives, avocadoes, olive oil and some cashews. Excellent, there you have four healthy fats!

3 › I'll leave dinner up to your creative freedom because, as I said, I don't want to give you a rigid eating model. So come on, make yourself something tasty and healthy.

With an efficient inclusion of healthy fats, without knowing it you will be ensuring that they become the leading stars of your diet. Yes, visually your plate will be full of vegetables of every color and they will dominate the "landscape" —good carbohydrates—. Next to them there will be a piece of beef, chicken or fish —the touch of protein—, but in the midst of all this there will be healthy fats in various forms —the masterstroke. And if we examine things from a nutritional intake point of view, what you will be consuming in the greatest quantity will be healthy fats. This is how to combine the three macronutrients in order to preserve your metabolic order.

I know that you like numbers, so I am going to give you some recommended proportions. Please calculate these percentages using your "eyemeter".

1 › Healthy fats should represent between 35 and 50 % of your dietary model (never less). That margin allows for a good intake.

2 › Proteins (animal or vegetable) should not be more than 20 % —that's how I work with my patients—. However, it's easier to find the proportion based on the clues I already gave you, taking into account your ideal body weight as a reference. I don't recommend a consumption of less than 0.8 grams per kilo of body weight, or more than two.

3 › The remaining percentage, depending on the quantity of healthy fats and proteins, is for vegetables, which you can eat care-free. Remember that the diets of all human beings should be rich in real plants.

4 › Putting it in clear numbers, if your percentage of healthy fats is 40 % and proteins is 20 %, the remaining 40 % is for carbohydrates (vegetables).

5 › Remember that this is not an exact science, don't drive yourself crazy making calculations, simply bear these instructions in mind and try to stick to these proportions, with the help of your common sense.

Fats are very versatile. They can be mixed with proteins —if you make a healthy mayonnaise, for example. You should use them to complement your vegetables— I have told you how —and, obviously, they can be your dessert. "Oh sure, doctor, I can drink a glass of olive oil and imagine it is dulce de leche!", you might want to angrily shout at me. Not at all. Buy dark chocolate with a cacao percentage no lower than 75 %, and take a good bite. Careful, not one of those candy bars which doesn't even contain cacao and which they sell in every corner of the supermarket —just read the list of ingredients on one of those products and start to panic—. At the end of the book I will share the recipe for one of my favorite desserts, which contains coconut milk, avocado and cacao, and I top it off with raspberries —it's top-notch—. Did you read that? You don't have to give up desserts. But you do have to give up those junk food options full of sucrose and chemicals which don't help your body in any way!

Why is a diet high in healthy fats recommended?

Because they provide many benefits for your organism —what a shame that Ancel Keys couldn't understand that—. While diets which are high in carbohydrates and low in fats are highly inflammatory (for the reasons you have read in this book), the opposite diets, high in healthy fats and low in carbs, especially when using fibrous carbohydrates such as vegetables —and with the help, on occasion, of resistant starches—, have proven to be highly protective of the metabolism, the cardiovascular system, brain, neurological, cognitive and anti-inflammatory functions, and contribute to hormonal development, among other benefits. This dietary system allows your body to use its accumulated fat as a primary energy source, without the help of energy bars, supplements or sweets which give your body cheap "gasoline" which doesn't last.

The Mediterranean diet, which has been used for centuries, is an example of this regime. Elsewhere there is the ketogenic diet —I introduced you to it in the second part of the book, the section about Charlie—, which finds its balance in 70 % fat, 20 % protein and 10 % carbohydrates. The ketogenic diet causes your body to produce so-called "ketone bodies", which are very good for the health of your brain and for controlling illnesses such as Parkinson's and Alzheimer's and hindering the life of cancer cells. I told you before and I repeat: the ketogenic diet is very demanding; if you don't follow it down to a T it won't work. If you eat a small piece of raspberry pie it will all have gone to pot, so, despite its benefits, I only recommend it to my patients with certain types of cancer, degenerative conditions, Parkinson's and epilepsy.

Of the three macronutrients, the fats are the ones which produce the quickest and longest-lasting feeling of fullness, another advantage! And, what's more, they are the ones which least stimulate the insulin. If you choose them well, if you use them without exception and in the correct measure, you will have taken an important step towards your healing. I tend to say to each of my patients: "Make your kitchen a restaurant and a drugstore", to create things which are delicious, full of flavor, a constant celebration, but also therapeutic. "But, doctor, I'm not sick". Well, exactly, to avoid getting ill.

However, don't lose sight of the fact that, for the sake of your metabolism, all three macronutrients are important, in the proportions we have already mentioned. I have seen to many patients who incorporate a good amount of healthy fats into their diet, consume the appropriate carbohydrates, but forget about the proteins, and obviously their organism experiences internal chaos. The protein intake should always be sufficient.

To sum up, and always bear this in mind...

It doesn't matter if you are a meat-eater, vegan, vegetarian, if you follow the "paleo" diet or the circus sword-swallowing diet, **if you want to correct your metabolism through your diet, be sure that it includes a good amount of healthy fats (more than 35 %), a controlled animal or vegetable protein intake (no greater than 20 %) and the remaining percentage set aside for carbohydrates (fibrous vegetables).** Remember that the proportion of protein that your organism needs is dependent on your ideal weight (according to your height) —I explained this not too long ago—. And, of course, it is necessary to have the results from your latest medical examinations, which give us clues as to how your metabolic indicators are doing: your lipid profile, and insulin, glucose, uric acid, thyroid, cortisol and leptin levels.

Bonus track

Many patients desperately ask me what they should do to keep following an appropriate diet when then go to a restaurant and they don't have all their oils, vegetables, nuts, vinegars and all of that by their side. I tend to give them this advice (I follow it when I go out to eat with Adriana and my young son). If you go to a restaurant with your partner, order a good piece of meat and share it; if you are a vegetarian, look for a plant protein option and order a big dish of vegetables, and share this too —like the Spanish tend to do, for example—. Ask the waiter to bring you some olive oil, ask him if they have any nuts, order a portion of avocado, add that to your vegetables, and there you have it. It is a simple way to keep your diet up. "Doctor, it's Saturday, and at that restaurant they sell that chocolate fondant I've told you so much about, it is unbeatable, spectacular…". Are you waiting for my approval? Eat it! And tomorrow get back to your routine. Give yourself permission every now and again. Don't be surprised if, one day, you lift your gaze to see me at the next table eating that same dessert. I also do it, in a controlled and responsible fashion. By the way, if you read this book, come over to my table and let me know if it helped you or not. I'd be very happy to hear it.

Chapter 11

When to eat

Doctor Jason Fung, who I greatly admire, tends to say that, firstly, "all diets work" and, secondly, "all diets fail". I couldn't be more in agreement with his assessment. You can do the most ridiculous diet in the world, like the pineapple diet, for example, and no doubt you will initially lose weight. You could obtain the same results with the redcurrant and oxygenated water diet, to name some nonsensical idea —"all diets work"—, but eventually, when your body gets used to it, you will gain weight again —"all diets fail"—. The same thing happens with the most well-planned, tailor-made, specialist and Ayurveda consultant-approved diet; even with the one I am proposing in this book. "What do you mean, doctor? So I wasted my money on *The metabolic miracle?*". No. I will explain in detail in this section.

The human body behaves the same way as business. The financial strategy which brought you good results last year most likely won't be successful over a five-year period. The same thing happens with our organism. You were overweight, had a disorder in your metabolism, but you started to apply the recommendations you read in this book. You took the tests, checked out your hormone levels, changed your diet —you made friends with lettuce—, included healthy fats, carbohydrates, the right protein, your life changed and, what's more, you lost weight. But after some time you felt as though your body started to put a few pounds back on. What happened, if you followed the plan down to a T, and it initially worked!? What happened is that, just like the financial strategy, it failed because it stayed the same. Your organism, which to begin with noticed the shake-up and was thankful for the change in habits, got used to it, got comfortable with it. There is a very famous quote that applies perfectly to this situation: "Insanity is doing the same thing over and over again and expecting different results". It is attributed to Albert Einstein but he never said it; whoever its creator was, they have my eternal thanks.

So what do you do when you feel like you have become "stagnant" and your healthy routines no longer work for you? Something very easy: invent a new financial strategy; in other words, shake your body off the routine and prepare yourself for the third step of your metabolic healing. The first step was learning what to leave out of your diet and what to include in it (relearning how to eat); the second was understanding how to combine all of these foods in order to control your metabolism. So, you stopped eating five or six times a day and opted for three —and you didn't die of starvation—. You left a window of five hours between breakfast, lunch and dinner, and you never ate the latter after 7:00 in the evening. You always had breakfast after 7:00 in the morning so that your body had rested for 12 hours without any food. Your insulin rested! Because the thing that most stimulates it is eating. Your liver worked the night shift and carried out gluconeogenesis! Your cortisol slept like a log! Furthermore, with all of those transformations, you taught your body to use its stored fat as its main source of energy. And you lost weight and everyone started to say: "You look really good!".

If you go over the process, you made some extremely valuable modifications and pulled your body out of its old routine. But after a while you started to notice that you had reached a limit, you weren't losing a pound, the scales even began to show a slight increase, and you shouted into the mirror: "I've hit a wall!". And you looked with mistrust at your lettuce, your coconut milk, your nuts and your extra virgin olive oil. It's normal: your organism, as a defense mechanism, will always try to get back to its previous weight, the one it knows, that weight you had for so many years, that fixed point known as set point. It's like the air-conditioning in hotels. It is programmed to maintain the temperature at 23 degrees Celsius —just an example—. If you open the window and the warm sea breeze flows in, the system will have to generate more cold air to compensate for the rise in temperature and return to those 23 degrees. Your body reacts in the same way. And that is the so-called set point, which also depends on two concepts which we addressed earlier: the basal metabolic rate and the energy expenditure in resting state, which the organism was used to for a long time.

There are two basic ways to get yourself out of this rut: 1) changing the frequency with which you eat and 2) changing the qualities of what you eat. Let's focus on the first one, frequency, which I will in turn divide into two moments: a) when to eat in a programmed manner and b) when to intuitively eat. This is the highest level of sophistication a human being can reach in terms of eating, it's the moment when you don't eat out of anxiety, impulse or cravings. But let's take a time out and carefully read the next paragraph.

This is a complex issue. In order to take this step, my first recommendation is this: ensure that you have indeed reached the "rut". If you are completely sure, do not advance without the advice of a professional. Why? Because the instructions for a fast are easy to identify, but only a specialist knows the contraindications. All human beings can fast, but not at every moment in our lives, and those moments can only be identified by an expert. Don't be swayed by the many bloggers and YouTubers who have irresponsibly turned fasting into a fad, without taking into account its adverse effects. It took me some time to understand it clearly. I managed to after having investigated in detail the world's dietary models, specializing in immunology and biochemistry and studying functional medicine, so as then to devote myself to functional nutrition and nutrigenomics. I'm talking about intermittent fasting, a term which a lot of people use without really knowing its meaning, its reach and its real benefits.

"No way, doctor. This really is the end of the world. Now you want me to nourish myself on air and that apple cider vinegar with The Mother thing?", you will complain, horrified. But it's not about that. When you looked at yourself in the mirror and said "I've hit a wall!", perhaps you didn't think about the main reason that happened: habit, routine, doing the same thing every day. So the time has come to vary the frequency with which you eat. But if you have got to that point, it is because you have done everything right (give yourself a point and a load of likes). Metabolic change is like a marathon: you have already run a good part of the race —in fact, you have modified your diet and your habits—; however, now you see a signpost in the road which says: "Turn left here".

As I was telling you, intermittent fasting has gained recognition because of influencers who want to turn it into a fashionable diet. What they, and most people, don't know is that fasting has always been a part of us. **Before we evolved into the homo iSapiens of social media, we were hunter-gatherers; if there was nothing to eat, our ancestors fasted. Food wasn't available all the time. Why didn't they die if they stopped feeding themselves for one,**

two, or even more days? I have told you several times in this book: the body, to make up for the absence of food, starts to produce energy from its stored fat. So our ancestors of many thousands of years ago fasted, and when they could hunt and eat, they celebrated. That's why it is despicable to me that some people label it the new slimming trend. Please, intermittent fasting is not new, it is not "fashionable" and it is not a "trend", it has always been an inherent part of being human, like walking or breathing.

You should fast

I will explain to you why it is worth doing, but if you feel ready to try it out, as well as reading these lines you should look for a specialist, a *certified* functional doctor who knows about functional nutrition in depth, or a doctor who is an expert on the topic, so that they can let you know if it really is in your interests to take this left turn, OK? What follows is understanding how you can pull your body out of its rut, its set point, and how you should begin fasting for 16, 24, 36 or 48 hours —again: always under the supervision of your specialist—.

Fasting should not be understood as a sacrifice or a religious act —although many communities from different religions do practice fasting—. Don't forget that many philosophers and thinkers have spoken about the mental clarity that comes from fasting and they don't get dizzy! I don't believe that God, the quantum field, chance, destiny, Buddha, the great energy or Elvis put us on this earth in order to eat every three hours. If that were meant to be our dietary regime, why then, with the exception of the countries along the equator, does the earth have seasons? Could our ancestors eat every day in winter?

I think this makes sense. If we look at it thoroughly from a bio-chemical perspective, if we go back to that "sermon" I gave you in the first pages of this book, the problem of metabolic syndrome diseases in the world, such as diabetes, high cholesterol and tri-glycerides, acne, obesity, high blood pressure and even infertility, is that they are caused by factors which stimulate inflammation in the body and by changes in the levels of insulin and friends. And what is it that stimulates insulin? Eating! Repeat with me: "Eating is what stimulates insulin".

That's why, if you decide *not* to eat, in a responsible, pro-grammed and guided manner, you can benefit your body by allowing the insulin to be on *off* mode. By not switching it on, after 24 or 36 hours of fasting you will have consumed the liver's glycogen levels and will access your fat and "burn" it —some call it fat "oxidation"—, if you have followed the correct steps laid out throughout this book.

Why is it called intermittent fasting? Because, as its name sug-gests, it gets interrupted, it gets started over, it changes. Let's su-ppose that you didn't listen to me and decided to take the leap, alone and with no parachute, into the land of fasting, with your own method called NMB (No More Breakfast). It was a Monday and you decided: "I am only going to eat twice a day, lunch and dinner". A short time afterwards, as your body has left its normal routine, you will lose weight, you will stop the rut. But if you conti-nue with the same regime, your organism will return to set point. Again, it will get used to it. It's like the example about a pay cut that we spoke about in the first part of the book. They can reduce your salary numerous times and you will always find a way to re-organize your spending. Here it applies in the same way. The body will always get used to living with the "salary" that we give it. Why did your creative NMB fast fail? Because it wasn't intermittent. It was always the same.

To get your body out of that set point, the fast needs to be varied. I am going to share my experience with this practice. When I know that one of those days which needs my full energy and mental clarity is coming up, I prefer not to eat. "For the love of God, doctor, how can you even think of that? Take care of yourself!". Thank you for thinking of me, but I do it with a full understanding of my body, consciously and voluntarily. I have trained my body for that. I have gone four days without eating. I have had week-long fasts and nothing has happened to me. I don't do it recklessly, I don't play with my health, I let my body take a rest from the act of eating for those days because I know the benefits of doing so. My body uses the energy from my fat; it is an extensive reserve, and, also, our organism, mine and yours, has protective mechanisms and starts to naturally produce the growth hormone in order to not "eat" the muscle. The practice of fasting, under these conditions, can be very beneficial for everyone, but it is necessary to understand its pros and cons, of which there are many, in depth.

Before asking my patients to start a 16, 24 or 36 hour fast if it's necessary, I get to know their cases really well. I know that their metabolism is under control, or at least that they are already in the process. Otherwise I would *never* recommend it as a *starter plan*. In fact, there are many contraindications and they aren't so easy to understand; for example, I don't recommend fasting to those who have some kind of metabolic condition relating to the adjustment of cortisol, because the period without eating will cause them stress and that will generate more cortisol, so it wouldn't have any kind of benefit for their metabolism. It is crucial to identify the reasons for prohibiting fasting or for knowing when to introduce it. I think that all human beings should fast. However, fasting is the same as garlic or coffee... yes, you already know the verse off by heart: fasting is good for all human beings —and we should practice it—, but not at every moment of our lives, due to its contraindications. However, once our metabolic disorders are corrected, we should *all* fast.

"But it should be totally forbidden for pregnant women, doctor!". How curious. During pregnancy it seems that everything is inadvisable. I am going to be very honest and a little out of order, but I think that the state in which women —intuitive by nature— are most connected with their bodies and its needs is during pregnancy. I experienced it with my wife. There are moments when they say: "No, I don't want to eat". And we shouldn't force them to. But, of course, then some family member, friend, or distant relative of Uncle Pete who is a pediatrician arrives and gives the standard sermon: "Don't be irresponsible, you are eating for two now, for you and your child!". And the poor pregnant woman, even though she knows that neither she nor her child need to, will eat. Why?

Fasting is not a trend. It is not new. It has always been with us. And, for metabolic control, it is, in my opinion, the best way to pull the body out of its routine. **If you are already dominating step one —what to eat and what not to eat— and step two —how to balance your food—, if you are already eating three times a day without sacrifices and letting your insulin rest for 12 hours after dinner, you could try not having breakfast for one or two days of the week and seeing how your body reacts. If you, dear reader, have not trained your organism with the indicated steps, please don't try it.**

I didn't write this chapter to convince you to fast. I wrote it so that you would know that you should fast if your body is ready. In this way you can keep quiet and just listen to your organism. Learn to hear it. So, when the time comes for one of your three meals, you will expertly know what to do. Silence. What is your body telling you? Have you noticed that the spirit which used to ask you for *pain au chocolat* with a double cappuccino is no longer there? Listen. Perhaps your organism will tell you it isn't hungry. It's likely. And if you don't have an appetite, even though it is breakfast time —for example—, don't eat. But don't do this to lose weight! Do it because, after all your training, you are ready to make this decision based on your intuition.

At the beginning of this section I spoke about the two paths to follow in order to drag your body out of its routine. We've looked at the first, varying the frequency with which you eat —intermittent fasting and intuitive fasting—; the second is changing the qualities of what you eat. How do you achieve that? This doesn't involve so many complications, but if you want to give it a go you must also have completed the two steps we have mentioned. If you already dominate them, **if you have your metabolism under control, then, using your eyemeter and common sense, vary the percentages of macronutrients a little. One day your diet can be higher in fats and lower in carbohydrates, the next day you can up the carbs and lower the fats; this is called *carbohydrate cycling*. With these variations you are stopping your body from getting used to the same thing.** This "cycling" works for some people and not for others; lots of people like it, others prefer not to do it. I recommend that, on the days which involve higher carbohydrates, you should include some kind of starch in one of your meals, such as potatoes, yucca or green plantain; or some kind of grain, like quinoa or brown rice. This way you will ensure that your dish has more carbs. The next day, remove these from your diet and, with that, you are varying your diet.

A very good strategy for patients who have their metabolism under control is to combine all of the aforementioned recommendations: intermittent fasting with carbohydrate cycling. That way you will mix the two variables: when to eat and the qualities of what you eat. If I had to choose, for me the intermittent fasting is much more powerful and closer to our nature and history. I can't stop thinking about our wise forefathers, sitting around the fire, eating the day's catch, focused on their food, enjoying it as if it were their last meal, not knowing if they would have any food tomorrow; not thinking about taking a photo of that big chunk of meat, or the fruits they collected that day, to upload onto Instagram. Fasting taught them something that we have lost, the celebration and gratitude for having food available.

Fasting heals

Finally, remember that you don't fast to try to make up for the poor information you have given your body with a bad diet. Fasting has to be a voluntary and conscientious act, a way of taking a moment's pause, of escaping the spiral of greed in a world which doesn't stop eating.

Its benefits for the metabolism are priceless: it will help to keep your body away from diabetes, fatty liver, polycystic ovaries and many types of infertility. It has positive mental and neurological effects, which are of great help with neurodegenerative, autoimmune and mitochondrial diseases; it also plays an important part in anti-aging, because it contributes to the modification of hundreds of genes which make us age quicker and in a worse way. It has an impact on concentration and learning; on meditation and contemplative states.

Investigators like Doctor Valter Longo —author of *The longevity diet*, 2017— have explained its benefits in reversing diseases like cancer, and have brought to light processes like autophagy, the body's capacity to eat itself. This isn't a mad, cannibalistic practice by our organism. It's quite the opposite. This process, mediated by the immune system and discovered by Japanese professor, Yoshinori Ohsumi —who received the Nobel Prize for Medicine in 2016 for this finding—, is responsible for selecting which cells your body needs and which it does not. Thus it promotes a sort of cellular renewal which is vital for your health and longevity. According to the studies of Longo and his team, this state is reached during prolonged fasting (around 48 hours).

A good way of simply explaining how fasting works in your body and how it contributes to controlling your metabolism is by using the following graphs. Remember all the concepts we have talked about and especially the behavior of our queen hormone, insulin. What is the only thing that stimulates her? Eating. If you eat all day, you are going to promote the formation of fat —unnecessary— in your body; whereas if you have periods without eating, your body will rest. Look at this diagram, which shows how insulin behaves inside any human being.

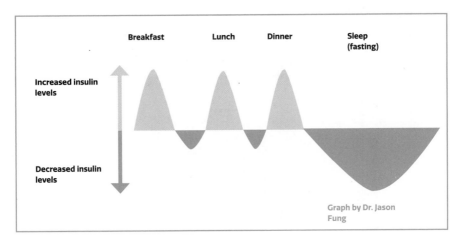

Graph by Dr. Jason Fung

Do you see? When you eat, your insulin levels rise. When the sugar from the food you have eaten stops being available in your blood, the insulin levels lower. This is the ideal blueprint: three meals a day. At night the royal hormone rests. Now look at what happens when you eat several times a day:

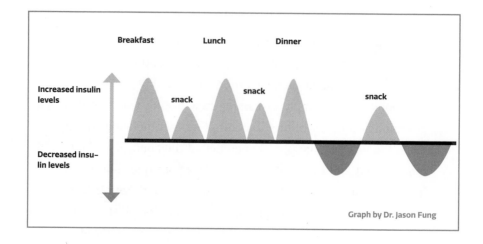

Graph by Dr. Jason Fung

Notice how the insulin almost never rests. Now think about the same blueprint with longer troughs and fewer peaks.

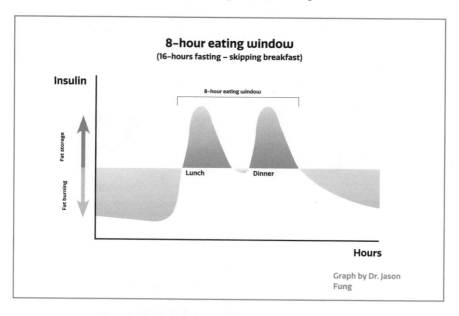

Graph by Dr. Jason Fung

Throughout all the periods when your insulin is at the metabolic spa taking a break, your organism will consume the glucose contained in the liver in the form of glycogen and then access its second turbine, the energy from fat, and start to "burn it".

You already know the answer

I know it has been a long journey, which began with the disheartening figures on the growth of metabolic syndrome diseases and the fatal victims they affect around the world. And here we are, coming up to the final phrases, and we end on the polar opposite, intermittent fasting. We have travelled from the irresponsible orgy of eating to the empty dish by choice. I hope that, after reading this book you have understood that those millions of deaths can be avoided with the best medicine of all, the one which is available every day at home: your food. What is food? Information. What type of information should you give your body? "Come on, doctor, there you go again with the endless questions. Well, we have to give it good information! Good food. Three times a day and without little containers, without powders, without little packets, without little desserts at breakfast". That's right! The solution is at the tip of your fork. Remember that. And if you forget something, go over it again, that's what this book is for. Use it as many times as you need to.

Feeding yourself well is the most powerful tool at your disposal, it is capable of modifying genes, inflammations and harmful processes in your body; eating badly will cause the exact opposite effect. Eating should always be an act of love and respect for yourself, for that temple which is your body. When you understand how to nourish yourself responsibly, you will be learning how to modify your entire interior universe, and that will reflect on the outside. Healthy eating brings us together, it gathers us around a table, it gives us a reason to celebrate. Conscientious nutrition should inspire us to join families and forever heal our communities.

At this very moment, a few lines before putting a final full stop to this book, I recall a conversation I had with my great teacher, Doctor Stanley Dudrick, creator of intravenous feeding, who I have mentioned several times in this book (a great of the medical world!). Having dinner at his house in Naugatuck (Connecticut) one day, I asked him about a topic which caused me plenty of concern: yes, science had made enormous strides in the nutrition of hospitalized patients, but poor diets were still killing millions of people around the world! "What can we do to improve this situation?", I asked him. He fell silent, stared at me, smiled and answered: "Carlos, I've already done my part, now you have to do yours. Go ahead". With this text that you hold in your hands, I have taken the first step, I have started to do "my part". That is what I dedicate and will dedicate my life to.

Now you might say: "Nice book, doctor, but what about the recipes you said you were going to give me? It's time to eat and I'm hungry". You're right. It's been a whole bunch of chapters talking about food; it's only fair that we try something healthy, nutritious and very tasty. In a couple of pages, I have several great options. "And is there a dessert, doctor?". Yes. A promise is a promise.

TEST
WHAT HAVE YOU LEARNT FROM THIS BOOK?

This is the end, or should I say, the beginning of your new dietary path and new lifestyle. If some of these questions raise doubts, well you know that you will find the answers in the previous pages. Do you accept your final metabolic mission? Answer this test.

1 › Can you eat everything in moderation?

2 › Are artificial sweeteners good because they don't contain calories?

3 › Do we need to exercise more and eat less?

4 › Is it worth counting how many calories you consume a day?

5 › If you opt for gluten-free bread, will you lose weight?

6 › Is it necessary to eat six times a day to maintain an active metabolism?

7 › Was the investigator Ancel Keys right about his theory on fats?

8 › Is salt bad and do we need to avoid it in our daily diet?

9 › If you don't eat at the same precise time and if you "skip" meals, will you get fat?

10 › Is breakfast the most important meal of the day?

11 › Are fats in our diet the cause of cardiac and circulatory diseases, and do saturated fats clog the arteries?

12 › Does eating an egg raise your cholesterol and is it equivalent to smoking a cigarette?

13 › Do you have to eat whenever your body "asks you to"?

14 › Should you consume several servings of fruit a day, and ideally between meals?

15 › Are fructose and agave syrup the ideal sweeteners for diabetics?

16 › Are fruit juices, and especially orange and mandarin, ideal for any person's diet?

17 › If you work out or exercise on an empty stomach, will you "eat" your muscles?

18 › Is a diet high in proteins and supplements the only way to have muscles like The Rock or Arnold Schwarzenegger?

19 › Do skinny people have a fast metabolism and fat people a slow metabolism?

20 › Are metabolic diseases hereditary and incurable?

21 › Do you have to consume a lot of sugar to give more gas to the body's tank?

22 › Are all calories the same, and do you have to be in a caloric deficit to be happy?

23 › Do children need sugar in their diet to give them the energy they need?

24 › Are lactose-free and fat-free milks better than whole milk?

25 › Do all human beings need dairy products to provide us with calcium so that our bones don't break?

RECISES

In collaboration with Denise Monroy
(@Denisemcook)

Let me make it clear that I am not a professional chef, but I am a cooking enthusiast. In fact, I am the one who cooks at home, and my wife is the one who washes the dishes and keeps me company while I invent something healthy and tasty to serve at the table.

I decided to include these recipes in *The metabolic miracle* to help you, dear reader, take your first steps towards a healthy diet. Here you will find a variety of options for breakfast, lunch and dinner. They are simple dishes, based on fresh and natural ingredients, and they don't contain sugar; sometimes we use stevia —make sure that yours is just that and not "sweetener *with* stevia"— but they do contain a lot of coconut, cacao, avocadoes, eggs, lots of vegetables, good oils and vinegars, good proteins —no tubs—, and they are prepared with lots of love, an added and entirely necessary ingredient!

Some of these dishes have been created in collaboration with my good friend, and fantastic chef, Denise Monroy (I recommend you follow her on Instagram: @Denisemcook); others were created by me, and some of them included the participation of Aunt Bertha —who, over the course of this book, has changed her diet—. You can find more recipes for you and your whole family on my website: drcarlosjaramillo.com.

And now... let's eat!

Breakfast

No-egg waffles

(1–2 servings)

....

INGREDIENTS

- 1 ½ CUPS HOMEMADE OR STORE-BOUGHT SUGAR-FREE COCONUT MILK

- 1 TABLESPOON APPLE VINEGAR

- ¼ CUP GHEE

- VANILLA TO TASTE

- 1 ¾ CUPS ALMOND OR COCONUT FLOUR

- ½ CUP OATS

- 1 ½ TEASPOONS BAKING POWDER

- A PINCH OF HIMALAYA SALT

- PECANS

- MACADAMIA BUTTER

METHOD AND SERVING

- Mix the coconut milk and apple vinegar and leave to rest for 5 minutes.
- Melt the ghee and mix with the vanilla and Himalaya salt.
- In a separate bowl, mix all the dry ingredients. Little by little, add the milk and vinegar mixture and the ghee mixture, and mix to form a smooth batter.
- Pour each serving into the waffle maker for around 5 minutes and leave to cook and crisp.
- For your topping, spread macadamia butter and sprinkle with pecans.

Omelet with eggplant, onion and basil

(1–2 SERVINGS)

INGREDIENTS

- 2 SCRAMBLED EGGS
- ½ EGGPLANT
- ¼ ONION
- COCONUT OIL
- FRESH BASIL
- PINK HIMALAYA SALT
- PEPPER
- OLIVE OIL

METHOD AND SERVING

- Sauté the eggplant and onion, chopped julienne, in coconut oil.
- Add the beaten eggs and cover for 5-7 minutes over a low heat.
- Top with the basil, pink Himalaya salt and pepper and drizzle olive oil over the omelet.

Chia pudding

(1–2 servings)

- 1 CUP SUGAR-FREE COCONUT MILK

- ½ CUP COCONUT CREAM

- 1 TEASPOON VANILLA (OPTIONAL)

- 1 TEASPOON STEVIA

- 3 TABLESPOONS ALMOND BUTTER

- ⅓ CUP CHIA SEEDS

- FRESH CRANBERRIES (OPTIONAL, FOR THE TOPPING)

METHOD AND SERVING

- In a blender on high speed, mix the coconut milk and cream, the stevia, 2 tablespoons of the almond butter and the vanilla (if using), to form a creamy mixture.
- Pour into a bowl and add the chia seeds and refrigerate for 30 minutes until they soak up the liquid.
- Before serving, mix well and leave to rest for 5 minutes.
- To serve, add another tablespoon of almond butter and the cranberries.

Avocado
and coconut *bowl*

(1–2 SERVINGS)

INGREDIENTS

- 2 LARGE HASS AVOCADOES

- ½ CUP SUGAR-FREE COCONUT MILK

- STEVIA TO TASTE

- 1 TEASPOON VANILLA EXTRACT

- A PINCH OF SALT

- 1 TABLESPOON CACAO NIBS

- 1 TABLESPOON DESICCATED COCONUT

- ¼ CUP MIXED BERRIES

- 1 TABLESPOON

WALNUTS

METHOD AND SERVING

- Blend the avocado, coconut milk, vanilla, stevia and salt to form a creamy mixture.
- Serve in a bowl and top with the cacao, the desiccated coconut, the berries and the walnuts.

"Rice" pudding

(2–4 SERVINGS)

INGREDIENTS

- 1 WHOLE CAULIFLOWER

- NATURAL COCONUT OR ALMOND MILK

- CINNAMON AND/OR CLOVES TO TASTE

- ORGANIC STEVIA DROPS

- 1 EGG WHITE FOR EVERY 2 CUPS OF COCONUT MILK (OPTIONAL)

- COCONUT CHIPS (OPTIONAL)

METHOD AND SERVING

- To remove the strong taste of the cauliflower, cook whole in plenty of water, bring to a boil, remove and leave to dry completely. You can do this the night before.

- In a saucepan, add one cup of coconut or almond milk per serving, 1 cup of grated cauliflower (which will look like rice) per serving, and cinnamon and/or cloves to taste.

- Cook over a medium heat to reduce the mixture.

- If using, add 1 egg white per 2 servings and cover, lowering the heat for a few minutes. Mix regularly. Leave to rest and add the stevia drops. This can be served hot or cold.

- Top with cranberries and cinnamon.

Baked eggs with romesco sauce

(4 SERVINGS)

Ingredients

- 8 FARM-FRESH EGGS
- 2 ½ RIPE TOMATOES
- ½ RED BELL PEPPER
- ½ CUP ALMONDS
- ½ CLOVE GARLIC
- ¼ CUP OLIVE OIL
- 5 BASIL LEAVES
- 2 DROPS STEVIA
- ¼ TEASPOON SEA SALT
- PEPPER TO TASTE
- ¼ CUP GREEK

Yogurt

Method and serving

- Preheat the oven to 200 °C.
- Place the tomatoes, sliced in half, in a baking tray with the almonds and garlic. Using a brush, spread with a little olive oil. Transfer to the oven for 35 minutes.
- Meanwhile, smoke the red pepper directly over a flame until it is totally black, leave to cool and then remove the skin and seeds.
- In a blender on medium speed, mix the red pepper, tomatoes, almonds, garlic, salt, basil, stevia and olive oil, until well mixed.
- In a deep oven dish, add the eggs, taking care not to break the yolks. Add 4 tablespoons of the sauce.
- Bake for 8 minutes at 200 °C until the eggs are cooked.
- Finish with pepper and a bit of Greek yogurt.

Main courses

Beef fillet with fresh salad

(2 SERVINGS)

INGREDIENTS

SALAD

- 4 MEDIUM BEETS

- 2 TABLESPOONS COCONUT OIL

- 1 SMALL WHITE ONION, CHOPPED

- 2 HASS AVOCADOES

- 10 MINT LEAVES

- 10 PEPPERMINT LEAVES

- ⅓ CUP CHOPPED CILANTRO

- 1 BUNCH ARUGULA

VINAIGRETTE

- ¼ CUP OLIVE OIL

- 2 TABLESPOONS CIDER VINEGAR

- 1 TEASPOON STEVIA

- 1 LARGE LEMON, THE JUICE

- 1 TEASPOON SEA SALT

Fillet

- 300 GR BEEF LOIN

- 1 TEASPOON PARSLEY

- 1 SMALL BUNCH FRESH ROSEMARY

- 1 SMALL BUNCH FRESH THYME

- SALT TO TASTE

- 1 TABLESPOON GRAPE SEED OIL

Method and serving

- Peel the beets and cut into pieces, massage with coconut oil and salt and place in the oven for 40 minutes at 200 °C.

- In a small bowl, thoroughly mix the olive oil, vinegar, lemon juice and stevia. Set aside.

- In a large bowl, mix the onion, beets, cilantro, mint, peppermint, avocado —diced— and arugula.

- Season and rub the fillet with the herbs and salt, chop into strips. Sauté the beef in a frying pan over medium heat; when it is still tender, remove from the heat and set aside for a few minutes.

- Serve the salad with the vinegar in a bowl and top with the beef strips.

Warm chicken breast, spinach and coconut salad

(2–3 SERVINGS)

INGREDIENTS

SALAD

- 1 ONION

- 1 LARGE GARLIC CLOVE

- ¼ TEASPOON SEA SALT

- 1 TABLESPOON GHEE, CLARIFIED BUTTER OR COCONUT OIL

- ¼ TEASPOON YELLOW MUSTARD SEEDS

- ¼ TEASPOON WHOLE CUMIN SEEDS

- ¼ TEASPOON PAPRIKA

- 1 CUP CARROTS (CHOPPED JULIENNE)

- 2 CUPS SPINACH, THOROUGHLY WASHED AND CHOPPED

- 1 LEMON, THE JUICE

- 1 ½ TABLESPOONS SUGAR-FREE DESICCATED COCONUT, LIGHTLY TOASTED

CHICKEN BREAST

- 1 BONELESS, SKINLESS CHICKEN BREAST

- 1 TABLESPOON MUSTARD

- 1 TABLESPOON MISO

- 1 TABLESPOON SALT

- ½ TABLESPOON GRAPE SEED OIL

- ⚜ On a chopping board, finely chop the onion and garlic. Place in a bowl and sprinkle with a bit of salt.
- ⚜ In a covered frying pan, heat the ghee and toast the mustard and cumin seeds for a few minutes. Add the paprika until it releases its aroma. Then, add the carrots, cook for approximately one more minute, then add the onion and garlic mixture and all the spinach. Keep stirring until the spinach begins to cook, about one minute.
- ⚜ Finish with a bit of lemon juice and the toasted coconut.
- ⚜ Cut the chicken into thin strips, rub with the Dijon mustard, miso and sea salt.
- ⚜ Place in a frying pan with a bit of oil over medium heat and leave for a few minutes until cooked.
- ⚜ Add to the salad and enjoy.

Vegetable curry

(4 SERVINGS)

INGREDIENTS

- ¾ CUP MUSHROOMS (CHOPPED)
- 1 SMALL SQUASH OR PUMPKIN (PEELED AND DICED)
- 3 TABLESPOONS COCONUT OIL
- 2 MEDIUM ONIONS (FINELY SLICED)
- 2 TABLESPOONS FRESH GINGER (GRATED)
- 2 CLOVES GARLIC (CHOPPED)
- 1 TABLESPOON MASALA CURRY POWDER
- 2 CUPS CAULIFLOWER (CHOPPED)
- 2 CANS COCONUT MILK
- 3-4 CUPS KALE OR SPINACH (CHOPPED)
- 2 TABLESPOONS FRESH LEMON JUICE
- ¼ CUP CASHEWS
- ½ CUP SPROUTS

METHOD AND SERVING

In a deep saucepan over medium heat, add the oil, onion, ginger and garlic. Sauté for 2 to 3 minutes, stirring constantly. Then add the curry powder and cook for 1 to 2 more minutes. Add the cauliflower and mushrooms and sauté until slightly golden. Add the coconut milk and stir to mix well. Lower the heat and cook for 5 minutes or so. Add the kale or spinach. Set aside.

In a baking tray, cook the squash with a bit of oil for 30 minutes at 250 °C. When ready, add to the curry mixture.

Serve in a bowl. Garnish with the cashews and sprouts, and add the lemon juice.

Salmon on broccoli *pesto*

(2 SERVINGS)

....

Ingredients

Pesto

- 1 LARGE BROCCOLI (ABOUT 2 CUPS)

- 2 BUNCHES FRESH BASIL OR SAGE

- ½ TABLESPOON LEMON

- ½ CUP ALMONDS

- 2 CLOVES GARLIC (CHOPPED)

- ½ CUP OLIVE OIL

- 2 TABLESPOONS WATER

- SALT AND PEPPER TO TASTE

Salmon

- 300 GRAMS SALMON FILLET, WITH OR WITHOUT SKIN

- 1 TABLESPOON LEMON JUICE

- 2-3 LARGE GARLIC CLOVES, GRATED

- ½ TEASPOON SALT

- ½ TEASPOON GROUND BLACK PEPPER

- 1-2 TEASPOONS AVOCADO OIL

- 2 SCALLIONS, FINELY SLICED

SALMON

- In a bowl, mix the lemon juice, garlic, salt and pepper
- Divide the salmon fillet into two portions and place in a large food storage bag with the previously prepared mixture. Seal the bag, attempting to remove as much air as possible. Gently move the fillets around the bag to ensure that they are uniformly covered in the mixture. Leave to marinate for 15 minutes, skin-side up.
- Preheat a frying pan over medium heat and add oil.
- Place the salmon fillets on the pan; when the skin is crispy, flip over and cook until the fillet is juicy in the center.

PESTO

- In a food processor, mix the broccoli, basil, almonds, garlic, oil and water, until forming a consistent texture.
- When the mixture is ready, add the lemon, salt and pepper. Mix well and set aside.
- Spread 4 tablespoons of the broccoli pesto on a plate and place the salmon fillet on top.

Carrot noodles with mushrooms

(2 SERVINGS)

Ingredients

SALAD

- 6 MEDIUM CARROTS (PEELED)

- ¼ CUP FRESH CILANTRO LEAVES

- 4 TEASPOONS TOASTED SESAME SEEDS

- 2 ONIONS (CHOPPED JULIENNE)

- 4 FINELY CHOPPED GARLIC CLOVES

- 350 GRAMS SHITAKE MUSHROOMS (CHOPPED)

- 400 GRAMS OYSTER MUSHROOMS OR PORTOBELLO MUSHROOMS (CHOPPED)

- 1 TEASPOON FRESH THYME

- 2 TABLESPOONS COCONUT OIL

- 2 FRESH BAY LEAVES

- 100 GRAMS WALNUTS

DRESSING

- THE ZEST OF ONE ORANGE

- 2 TABLESPOONS LEMON JUICE

- 4 TABLESPOONS OLIVE OIL

- 2 TABLESPOONS TOASTED SESAME SEEDS

- SEA SALT

- FRESHLY GROUND BLACK PEPPER

SALAD

- ❧ Using a mandolin or noodle maker, cut the carrots into long, thin strips, like spaghetti (or as you prefer). In a bowl, mix the carrot, cilantro leaves and sesame seeds. Set aside.
- ❧ Heat the oil in a large frying pan over medium heat, add the onion and garlic and cook for 3 minutes, and then add the mushrooms, thyme and bay leaves and stir constantly for about 10 minutes or until the mushrooms release their juices.
- ❧ Add the walnuts and the carrot mixture.

DRESSING

- ❧ Using a hand mixer, mix the orange zest, lemon juice, olive oil, sesame seeds, salt and pepper, until forming a uniform mixture.
- ❧ To serve, add the dressing to the carrot salad to taste.

Green burritos with mushroom and nut 'meat'

(4 SERVINGS)

INGREDIENTS

MUSHROOM AND NUT MEAT

- 1 CUP SHITAKE MUSHROOMS (CHOPPED)

- 5 RED TOMATOES

- 1 CUP WALNUTS (CHOPPED)

- 1 MEDIUM CAULIFLOWER (CHOPPED)

- 2 CLOVES GARLIC (CHOPPED)

- 2 TABLESPOONS OLIVE OIL

- ½ TEASPOON SEA SALT

- 1 TABLESPOON SMOKED PAPRIKA

- 1 TABLESPOON GROUND CUMIN

- 1 TABLESPOON

CHILI POWDER

- 1 SPRIG THYME

- 5 DROPS STEVIA

- 1 TEASPOON SEA SALT

CASHEW CREAM

- 1 ½ CUPS RAW CASHEWS (SOAKED)

- 1 CUP WATER

- ½ TEASPOON SEA SALT

- ¼ TEASPOON GARLIC POWDER

- ½ TEASPOON CUMIN POWDER

- 1 PINCH CHILI POWDER

- 1 CHIPOTLE SOAKED IN HOT WATER

- 1 TABLESPOON OLIVE OIL

Burrito assembly

- ½ AVOCADO, SLICED

- CILANTRO TO TASTE

- RED ONION TO TASTE

- 8 LETTUCE LEAVES

- 1 TEASPOON LEMON JUICE

Method and serving

Mushroom and nut meat

- Grate the tomatoes until you get out all the pulp. Set aside.
- In a frying pan, sauté the garlic, cauliflower and mushrooms, and cook over a medium heat until the cauliflower starts to brown; add the chopped nuts, grated tomato, ground cumin, chili and thyme, and cook for a few minutes.
- Add salt and stevia.

Cashew cream

- Place all of the ingredients in a blender and mix until forming a completely creamy mixture.
- Serve in a separate bowl.

Burrito assembly

- Top a lettuce leaf with two tablespoons of nut meat, the avocado, one tablespoon of cashew cream, cilantro, onion and a couple of drops of lemon.
- Place all the ingredients in the center of the lettuce leaf, roll it up as if it were a burrito and enjoy!

Desserts

Raw carrot cake with cashew frosting

Ingredients

Frosting

- 2 CUPS CASHEWS, SOAKED PREVIOUSLY

- 2 TEASPOONS LEMON

- 2 TEASPOONS COCONUT OIL

- 1 DATE (OPTIONAL)

- WATER, AS NEEDED

Cake

- 2 GROUND OR GRATED CARROTS (NOT BLENDED)

- 1 ½ CUPS GLUTEN-FREE WHOLE OATS

- ½ CUP DATES

- 1 CUP SUGAR-FREE DESICCATED COCONUT

- 1 TEASPOON CINNAMON POWDER

- 3 TEASPOONS COCONUT OIL

METHOD

FROSTING

- ❧ Place all the ingredients in a blender and add water.
- ❧ Blend until forming a thick texture.

CAKE

- ❧ Grind all of the ingredients (do not blend) and mix until forming a smooth dough.
- ❧ Add half the dough to a recipient and apply pressure to compact into the bottom layer. Add some frosting and freeze for an hour.
- ❧ Compact a second layer of dough on top and refrigerate for another hour.
- ❧ Remove from the mold and add the rest of the frosting.
- ❧ Grate some lemon zest on top.

Truffles

COCONUT

- 250 TO
  300 GRAMS
  CHOCOLATE,
  MINIMUM 85 %
  CACAO

- ¼ CUP COCONUT
  OIL

- ¾ CUP WHOLE
  COCONUT MILK

- ¼ TEASPOON SEA
  SALT

- VANILLA TO
  TASTE

- COCOA POWDER
  AND CHOPPED

METHOD

- Cook the chocolate and coconut oil in a bain marie until forming a uniform mixture.
- Add coconut milk and remove from the heat. Mix until forming a consistent mixture.
- Add salt and vanilla (optional).
- Refrigerate for 1-2 hours. Then, make portions using a spoon and form into balls or squares with your hands. Roll in the cocoa powder or chopped coconut.
- Refrigerate for another 15 minutes.
- Store in a cool place.

Chocolate mousse

Ingredients

- 2 Eggs

- 1 Bar (80 to 100 Grams) Chocolate, Minimum 85 % Cacao

Method

- Separate the egg yolks and whites
- Whisk the egg whites to stiff peaks.
- Separately, beat the yolks.
- Melt the chocolate in a bain marie.
- Add the melted chocolate to the yolks and mix.
- Little by little, add the egg whites and keep mixing to form a uniform mixture.
- Refrigerate for 4 hours and decorate to taste.

ACKNOWLEDGEMENTS

Above all, thanks to you, dear reader, for buying this book, the first of many I hope to write.

Thanks to Planeta publishing house and my editor, Marcela Riomalo, who firmly believed in this project. Thanks to Patxo Escobar, with whom I shared dinners, a couple of single malts and exchanged millions of emails, calls and WhatsApp messages, even at unearthly hours, to fine tune the writing of this text; in the process, I gained a good friend —and I'm happy to know that he has put many of this book's teachings into practice—.

Thanks to my faithful dog, Toña, who was witness to my hours of reading and writing to put together these chapters. She is now gone, she said her goodbyes to us as I was finishing this book.

Thanks to God, to my parents, my cousin and my friends who have always believed in me (you know who you are).

And, last but not least, my infinite thanks to my wife, Adriana, my greatest life choice; the person who has always supported me, trusted me, been at my side for all my projects, and who read the drafts of the chapters I was writing about three thousand times —she was my in-house editor—. By her side and from our home, with our son Luciano and our little bulldog Rocco, I feel like anything is possible.

puccini.

Bibliography

Part one
The metabolic problem

Chapter 1
The epidemic

- World Health Organization. Global report on diabetes. 2016. Available at https://apps.who.int/iris/bitstream/handle/10665/204871/9789241565257_eng.pdf. Consulted June 6, 2017.
- Centers for Disease Control and Prevention. Number (in Millions) of Civilian, Non-Institutionalized Persons with Diagnosed Diabetes, United States, 1980-2014. Available at: https://www.cdc.gov/diabetes/statistics/prev/national/figpersons.htm. Consulted June 6, 2017. Used with permission.
- Tabish, S. A. Is diabetes becoming the biggest epidemic of the twenty-first century? Int J Health Sci. 2007;1(2):5-8.
- Yudkin, J. Diet and coronary thrombosis hypothesis and fact. Lancet. 27 July, 1957;273(6987):155-162.
- Yudkin, J. The causes and cure of obesity. Lancet. 19 December, 1959;274(7112):1135-1138.
- Xu, Y. et al. Prevalence and Control of Diabetes in Chinese adults. JAMA. 2013;310(9):948-958.
- Menke, A. et al. Prevalence of and trends in diabetes among adults in the United States, 1988–2012. JAMA. 2015;314(10):1021-1029.

- Polonsky, K. S. The past 200 years in diabetes. N Engl J Med 2012;367(14):1332-1340.
- National Heart, Lung, and Blood Institute [Internet]. Maintaining a healthy weight on the go. April 2010. Available at: nhlbi.nih.gov/health/public/heart/obesity/aim_hwt.pdf.

Chapter 2
The big lie

- Brownell, K. D., Puhl, R. M., Schwartz, M. B. y L. Rudd (eds.). (2005). Weight bias: Nature, consequences, and remedies. New York, NY: Guilford Publications.
- Ludwig, D. S. Weight loss strategies for adolescents: A 14-year-old struggling to lose weight. JAMA. February 1, 2012;307(5):498-508.
- Ebbeling, C. B., Swain, J. F., Feldman, H. A., Wong, W. W., Hachey, D. L., Garcia-Lago, E. y D. S. Ludwig. Effects of dietary composition on energy expenditure during weight-loss maintenance. JAMA. June 27, 2012;307(24):2627-2634. doi: 10.1001/jama.2012.6607. PubMed [citation] PMID: 22735432, PMCID: PMC3564212.
- Suminthran, P. Long-term persistence of hormonal adaptations to weight loss. N Engl J Med. October 27, 2011;365(17):1597-1604.
- Keys, A., Brožek, J., Henschel, A., Mickelsen, O. y H. L. Taylor. The biology of human starvation (2 volumes). MINNE ed. St. Paul, MN: University of Minnesota Press; 1950.
- O'Meara, S., Riemsma, R., Shirran, L., Mather, L. y G. Ter Riet GA systematic review of the clinical effectiveness of orlistat used for the management of obesity. Obes Rev. February 2004;5(1):51-68.

- Torgerson, J. S. et al. Xenical in the Prevention of Diabetes in Obese Subjects (XENDOS) Study. Diabetes Care. January 2004;27(1):155-161.

- Ladabaum, U. et al. Obesity, abdominal obesity, physical activity, and caloric intake in US adults: 1988 to 2010. Am J Med. August 2014;127(8):717-727.

- Sims, E. A. Experimental obesity in man. J Clin Invest. Mayo de 1971;50(5):1005-1011.

- Sims, E. A. et al. Endocrine and metabolic effects of experimental obesity in man. Recent Prog Horm Res. 1973;29:457-496.

- Shell E. R. The hungry gene: the inside story of the obesity industry. New York: Grove Press; 2003.

- Countries that exercise the most include United States, Spain, and France. Huffington Post [Internet]. December 31, 2013. Available at: huffingtonpost.ca/2013/12/31/country-exercise-most-_n_4523537.html. Consulted April 6, 2015.

- Dwyer-Lindgren, L., Freedman, G., Engell, R. E., Fleming, T. D., Lim, S. S., Murray, C. J. and A. H. Mokdad. Prevalence of physical activity and obesity in US counties, 2001–2011: A road map for action. Population Health Metrics. July 10, 2013;11:7. Available at: biomedcentral.com/content/pdf/1478-7954-11-7. pdf. Consulted April 8, 2015.

Chapter 3
What makes us sick

- Guyton and Hall Textbook of Medical Physiology, 13th edition, 2016.

- Smith, C. J., Fisher, M. y G. A. McKay,. Drugs for diabetes: part 2 sulphonylureas. Br J Cardiol. November 2010;17(6):279-282.

- Domecq, J. P. et al. Drugs commonly associated with weight change: A systematic review and meta-analysis. J Clin Endocrinol Metab. February 2015;100(2):363-370.

- Kong, L. C. et al. Insulin resistance and inflammation predict kinetic body weight changes in response to dietary weight loss and maintenance in overweight and obese subjects by using a Bayesian network approach. Am J Clin Nutr. December 2013;98(6):1385-1394.

- Martin, S. S., Qasim, A. and M. P. Reilly. Leptin resistance: A possible interface of inflammation and metabolism in obesity-related cardiovascular disease. J Am Coll Cardiol. October 7, 2008;52(15):1201-1210.

- Lustig, R. H. et al. Obesity, leptin resistance, and the effects of insulin suppression. Int J Obesity. August 17, 2004;28:1344-1348.

- Fauci, A. et al., eds. Harrison's principles of internal medicine. 17.ª ed. McGraw-Hill Professional; 2008. P. 2255.

- Hirsch, K. R., Smith-Ryan, A. E., Blue, M. N. M., Mock, M. G. and E. T. Trexler. Influence of segmental body composition and adiposity hormones on resting metabolic rate and substrate utilization in overweight and obese adults. J Endocrinol Invest. June 2017;40(6):635-643. doi: 10.1007/s40618-017-0616-z. Electronic publication: February 16, 2017.

- Yamanaka, Y., Motoshima, H. and K. Uchida. Hypothalamic-pituitary-adrenal axis differentially responses to morning and evening psychological stress in healthy subjects. Neuropsychopharmacol Rep. November 27, 2018. doi: 10.1002/ npr2.12042.

- Jensen, T., Niwa, K., Hisatome, I., Kanbay, M., Andrés-Hernando, A., Roncal-Jiménez, C. A., Sato, Y., García, G., Ohno, M., Lanaspa, M. A., Johnson, R. J. and M. Kuwabara. Increased Serum Uric Acid over five years is a Risk Factor for Developing Fatty Liver. Sci Rep. August 6, 2018;8(1):11735. doi: 10.1038/s41598-018-30267-2.

- Kuwabara, M., Kuwabara, R., Niwa, K., Hisatome, I., Smits, G., Roncal-Jiménez, C. A., MacLean, P. S., Yracheta, J. M., Ohno, M., Lanaspa, M. A., Johnson R. J. and D. I. Jalal. Different Risk for Hypertension, Diabetes, Dyslipidemia, and Hyperuricemia According to Level of Body Mass Index in Japanese and American Subjects. Nutrients. August 3, 2018;10(8).

- King, C., Lanaspa, M. A., Jensen, T., Tolan, D. R., Sánchez-Lozada, L. G. and R. J. Johnson. Uric Acid as a Cause of the Metabolic Syndrome. Contrib Nephrol. 2018;192:88-102. doi: 10.1159/000484283. Electronic publication: January 23, 2018.

- Johnson, R. J., Sánchez-Lozada, L. G., Andrews, P. and M. A. Lanaspa. Perspective: A Historical and Scientific Perspective of Sugar and Its Relation with Obesity and Diabetes. Adv Nutr. May 15, 2017;8(3):412-422. doi: 10.3945/an.116.014654. Print version: May 2017.

- Johnson, R. J., Nakagawa, T., Sánchez-Lozada, L. G., Shafiu, M., Sundaram, S., Le, M., Ishimoto, T., Sautin, Y. Y. and M. A. Lanaspa. Sugar, uric acid, and the etiology of diabetes and obesity. Diabetes. October 2013;62(10):3307-3315. doi: 10.2337/db12-1814.

- Lanaspa, M. A., Sánchez-Lozada, L. G., Choi, Y. J., Cicerchi, C., Kanbay, M., Roncal-Jiménez, C. A., Ishimoto, T., Li, N., Marek, G., Duranay, M., Schreiner, G., Rodríguez-Iturbe, B., Nakagawa, T., Kang, D. H., Sautin, Y. Y. and R. J. Johnson. Uric acid induces hepatic steatosis by generation of mitochondrial oxidative stress: Potential role in fructose-dependent and-independent fatty liver. J Biol Chem. November 23, 2010;287(48):40732-40744. doi: 10.1074/jbc.M112.399899. Electronic publication: October 3, 2010. PMID: 23035112

Chapter 4
Anxiety and
food addiction

- Nutt, D. Development of a rational scale to assess the harm of drugs of potential misuse. Lancet. March 24, 2007;369(9566):1047-1053.
- Gearhardt, A. N.Food addiction: An examination of the diagnostic criteria for dependence. J Addict Med. March 2009;3(1):1-7.
- Colantuoni, C. Excessive sugar intake alters binding to dopamine and mu-opioid receptors in the brain. Neuroreport. November 16, 2001;12(16):3549-3552.
- Volkow, N. D. "Nonhedonic" food motivation in humans involves dopamine in the dorsal striatum and methylphenidate amplifies this effect. Synapse. June 1, 2002;44(3):175-180.
- Lenoir, M. Intense sweetness surpasses cocaine reward. PLoS One. August 1, 2007;2(8):e698.
- Wang, Y. C., Bleich, S. N. and S. L. Gortmaker. Increasing caloric contribution from sugar-sweetened beverages and 100 % fruit juices among US children and adolescents, 1988-2004. Pediatrics. June 2008;121(6):e1604-1614. doi: 10.1542/peds.2007-2834.
- Fung, T. T. Sweetened beverage consumption and risk of coronary heart disease in women. Am J Clin Nutr. April 2009;89(4):1037-1042. doi: 10.3945/ajcn.2008.27140. Electronic publication: February 11, 2009.
- Malik, V. S. Intake of sugar-sweetened beverages and weight gain: A systematic review. Am J Clin Nutr. August 2006;84(2):274-288.
- Forshee, R. A. Sugar-sweetened beverages and body mass index in children and adolescents: A meta-analysis. Am J Clin

Nutr. June 2008;87(6):1662-1671. Errata in: Am J Clin Nutr. January 2009;89(1):441-442.

- Wang, Y. C. and D. S. Ludwig. Impact of change in sweetened caloric beverage consumption on energy intake among children and adolescents. Arch Pediatr Adolesc Med. April 2009;163(4):336- 343. doi: 10.1001/archpediatrics.2009.23.

- Ludwig, D. S. Artificially sweetened beverages: Cause for concern. JAMA. December 9, 2009;302(22):2477-2478. doi: 10.1001/jama.2009.1822.

Chapter 5
Chronic inflamm

- Deng, Y. Adipokines as novel biomarkers and regulators of the metabolic syndrome. Ann N Y Acad Sci. November 2010;1212:E1-E19. doi: 10.1111/j.1749-6632.2010.05875.x

- Nimptsch, K., Konigorski, S., and T. Pischon, Diagnosis of obesity and use of obesity biomarkers in science and clinical medicine. Metabolism. December 23, 2018. pii: S0026-0495(18)30266-X. doi: 10.1016/j.metabol.2018.12.006 [Electronic publication before print].

- Jones, O. A., Maguire, M. L. and J. L. Griffin. Environmental pollution and diabetes: A neglected association. Lancet. January 26, 2008;371(9609):287-288. doi: 10.1016/S0140-6736(08)60147-6.

- Atkinson, R. L. Viruses as an etiology of obesity. Mayo Clin Proc. October 2007;82(10):1192-1198.

- Shamriz, O. and Y. Shoenfeld. Infections: A double-edge sword in autoimmunity. Curr Opin Rheumatol. July 2018;30(4):365- 372.

- Ram, R. and G. Morahan. Effects of Type 1 Diabetes Risk Alleles on Immune Cell Gene Expression. Genes (Basel). January 21, 2017;8(6). ▪

- Yuan, Y. Obesity-Related Asthma: Immune Regulation and Potential Targeted Therapies. J Immunol Res. June 28, 2018;2018:1943497.

- Carpaij, O. A. and M. van den Berge. The asthma-obesity relationship: Underlying mechanisms and treatment implications. Curr Opin Pulm Med. January 2018;24(1):42-49.

- Nirmalkar, K. Gut Microbiota and Endothelial Dysfunction Markers in Obese Mexican Children and Adolescents. Nutrients. December 19, 2018;10(12).

- Bohan, R. Gut microbiota: A potential manipulator for host adipose tissue and energy metabolism. J Nutr Biochem. November 10, 2018;64:206-217.

- Belizário, J. E. and J. Faintuch. Microbiome and Gut Dysbiosis. Exp Suppl. 2018;109:459-476.

- Wilders, M. IgG antibodies against food antigens are correlated with inflammation and intima media thickness in obese juveniles. Exp Clin Endocrinol Diabetes. April 2008;116(4):241-245.

- DiNicolantonio, J. J. and J. H. O'Keefe. Importance of maintaining a low omega-6/omega-3 ratio for reducing inflammation. Open Heart. November 26, 2018;5(2).

- Khadge, S. Immune regulation and anti-cancer activity by lipid inflammatory mediators. Int Immunopharmacol. December 2018;65:580-592.

- Holick, M. F. Vitamin D: Importance in the prevention of cancers, type 1 diabetes, heart disease, and osteoporosis. Am J Clin Nutr. March 2004;79(3):362-371.

- Darroudi, S. Oxidative stress and inflammation, two features associated with a high percentage body fat, and that may lead to diabetes mellitus and metabolic syndrome. Biofactors. December 18, 2018.

- Battelli, M. G. Metabolic syndrome and cancer risk: The role of xanthine oxidoreductase. Redox Biol. December 7, 2018;21.

- De Jongh, R. T., van Schoor, N. M. and P. Lips. Changes in vitamin D endocrinology during aging in adults. Mol Cell Endocrinol. September 15, 2017;453:144-150.

- Mazidi, M., Michos, E. D. and M. Banach. The association of telomere length and serum 25-hydroxyvitamin D levels in US adults: The National Health and Nutrition Examination Survey. Arch Med Sci. February 1, 2017;13(1):61-65.

- Marcon, F. Telomerase activity, telomere length and hTERT DNA methylation in peripheral blood mononuclear cells from monozygotic twins with discordant smoking habits. Environ Mol Mutagen. October 2017;58(8):551-559.

- Malhotra, A. Saturated fat does not clog the arteries: Coronary heart disease is a chronic inflammatory condition, the risk of which can be effectively reduced from healthy lifestyle interventions. Br J Sports Med. August 2017;51(15):1111-1112. doi: 10.1136/bjsports-2016-097285. Electronic publication: April 25, 2017.

Part two
Metabolic myths

Chapter 6
Foodstuffs

Proteins

- Yin, J. Protein restriction and cancer. Biochim Biophys Acta Rev Cancer. April 2018;1869(2):256-262. doi: 10.1016/j.bbcan.2018.03.004. Electronic publication: March 26, 2018.

- Stojkovic, V. The Effect of Dietary Glycemic Properties on Markers of Inflammation, Insulin Resistance, and Body Composition in Postmenopausal American Women: An Ancillary Study from a Multicenter Protein Supplementation Trial. Nutrients. May 11, 2017;9(5). pii: E484. doi: 10.3390/ nu9050484.

- Calton, E. K. Certain dietary patterns are beneficial for the metabolic syndrome: reviewing the evidence. Nutr Res. July 2014;34(7):559-568. doi: 10.1016/j.nutres.2014.06.012. Electronic publication: June 26, 2014.

- Bouvard, V., Loomis, D., Guyton, K. Z. et al. Carcinogenicity of consumption of red and processed meat. Lancet Oncol. December 2015;16(16):1599-1600.

- Alexander, D. D. and C. A. Cushing. Red meat and colorectal cancer: A critical summary of prospective epidemiologic studies. Obes Rev. May 2011 May;12(5):e472-e493.

- Lin, J., Zhang, S. M., Cook, N.R. et al. Dietary fat and fatty acids and risk of colorectal cancer in women. Am J Epidemiol. November 15, 2004;160(10):1011-1022.

- Sapkota, A. R., Lefferts, L. Y., McKenzie, S. et al. What do we feed to food-production animals? A review of animal feed ingredients and their potential impacts on human health. Environ Health Perspect. May 2007;115(5):663-670.

- Centers for Disease Control and Prevention. Salmonella and chicken: what you should know and what you can do. https://www.cdc.gov/features/SalmonellaChicken/index.html. Updated September 11, 2017.
- Food and Drug Administration. Department of Health and Human Services. 2012 Summary Report on Antimicrobials Sold or Distributed for Use in Food-Producing Animals. https://www.fda.gov/downloads/ForIndustry/UserFees/AnimalDrugUserFeeActADUFA/UCM416983.pdf. September 2014.
- Consumer Reports. Dangerous contaminated chicken. http://www.consumerreports.org/cro/magazine/2014/02/the-highcost-of-cheap-chicken/index.htm. Updated January 2014.
- Klein, S., Witmer, J., Tian, A. and C. S. deWaal. Center for Science in the Public Interest. The Ten Riskiest Foods Regulated by the U.S. Food and Drug Administration. October 7, 2009.
- Johns Hopkins Bloomberg School of Public Health. Global shift in farmed fish feed may impact nutritional benefits ascribed to consuming seafood. http://www.jhsph.edu/research/centers-and-institutes/johns-hopkins-center-for-a-livable-future/news-room/ News-Releases/2016/global-shift-in-farmed-fish-feed-may-impact-nutritional-benefits-ascribed-to-consuming-seafood.html. March 14, 2016.
- Done, H. Y. and R. U. Halden. Reconnaissance of 47 antibiotics and associated microbial risks in seafood sold in the United States. J Hazard Mater. June 23, 2015;282:10-17.
- Fry, J. P., Love, D. C., MacDonald, G. K. et al. Environmental health impacts of feeding crops to farmed fish. Environ Int. May 2016;91:201-214.

- Mozaffarian, D. and E. B. Rimm. Fish intake, contaminants, and human health: evaluating the risks and the benefits. JAMA. 2006;296(15):1885-1899.

- Del Gobbo L, C., Imamura, F., Aslibekyan, S. et al. Ω-3 Polyunsaturated fatty acid biomarkers and coronary heart disease: Pooling project of 19 cohort studies. JAMA Intern Med. August 1, 2016;176(8):1155-1166.

- Whiteley, P. Gluten- and casein-free dietary intervention for autism spectrum conditions. Front Hum Neurosci. January 4, 2013;6:344. doi: 10.3389/fnhum.2012.00344. eCollection 2012.

Fats

- Siri-Tarino, P. W., Sun, Q., Hu, F. B. et al. Saturated fat, carbohydrate, and cardiovascular disease. Am J Clin Nutr. 2010;91(3):502- 509.

- Volk, B. M., Kunces, L. J., Freidenreich, D. J. et al. Effects of step-wise increases in dietary carbohydrate on circulating saturated fatty acids and palmitoleic acid in adults with metabolic syndrome. PLoS One. November 21, 2014;9(11):e113605.

- Chowdhury, R., Warnakula, S., Kunutsor, S. et al. Association of dietary, circulating, and supplement fatty acids with coronary risk: a systematic review and meta-analysis. Ann Intern Med. March 18, 2014;160(6):398-406.

- Aarsland, A. and R. R. Wolfe. Hepatic secretion of VLDL fatty acids during stimulated lipogenesis in men. J Lipid Res. 1998;39(6):1280-1286.

- Lorente-Cebrián, S., Costa, A.G., Navas-Carretero, S. et al. Role of omega-3 fatty acids in obesity, metabolic syndrome, and cardiovascular diseases: A review of the evidence. J Physiol Biochem. September 2013;69(3):633–651.

- Carrie, L., Abellan van Kan, G., Rolland, Y. et al. PUFA for prevention and treatment of dementia? Curr Pharm Des. 2009;15(36):4173-4185.

- Loef, M. and H. Walach. The omega-6/omega-3 ratio and dementia or cognitive decline: A systematic review on human studies and biological evidence. J Nutr Gerontol Geriatr. 2013;32(1):1-23.

- Hibbeln, J. R. Depression, suicide and deficiencies of omega-3 essential fatty acids in modern diets. World Rev Nutr Diet. 2009;99:17-30.

- Simopoulos, A. P. The importance of the ratio of omega-6/omega-3 essential fatty acids. Biomed Pharmacother. October 2002;56(8):365-379.

- Eades, M. The Blog of Michael R. Eades, M.D. [Internet]. Framingham follies. September 28, 2006. Available at: proteinpower.com/drmike/cardiovascular-disease/framingham-follies.

- Howard, B. V. et al. Low fat dietary pattern and risk of cardiovascular disease: The Womens' Health Initiative Randomized Controlled Dietary Modification Trial. JAMA. February 8, 2006;295(6):655-666.

- Willett, W. C. Dietary fat plays a major role in obesity: No. Obes Rev. May 2002;3(2):59-68.

- Sacks, F. M. et al. American Heart Association. Dietary Fats and Cardiovascular Disease: A Presidential Advisory from the American Heart Association. Circulation. July 18, 2017;136(3):e1-e23.

- Malhotra, A. Saturated fat does not clog the arteries: Coronary heart disease is a chronic inflammatory condition, the risk of which can be effectively reduced from healthy lifestyle interventions. Br J Sports Med August 2017;51(15):1111-1112.

doi: 10.1136/bjsports-2016-097285. Electronic publication: April 25, 2017.

- Ramsden, C. E. et al. Re-evaluation of the traditional die-theart hypothesis: Analysis of recovered data from Minnesota Coronary Experiment (1968-1973). BMJ. April 12, 2016;353:i1246.

- Dehghan, M., Mente, A. Zhang, X. et al. Associations of fats and carbohydrate intake with cardiovascular disease and mortality in 18 countries from five continents (PURE): A prospective cohort study. Lancet. August 29, 2017.

- Masterjohn, C. Saturated fat does a body good. Weston A. Price Foundation. May 6, 2016.

- National Cholesterol Education Program Expert Panel on Detection, Evaluation, and Treatment of High Blood Cholesterol in Adults (Adult Treatment Panel III). National Institutes of Health; National Heart, Lung, and Blood Institute. September 2002. Available at: nhlbi.nih.gov/files/docs/resources/heart/ atp3full.pdf. Consulted April 12, 2015.

- Siri-Tarino, P. W. et al. Meta-analysis of prospective cohort studies evaluating the association of saturated fat with cardiovascular disease. Am J Clin Nutr. March 2010;91(3):535-546.

- Yamagishi, K. et al. Dietary intake of saturated fatty acids and mortality from cardiovascular disease in Japanese. Am J Clin Nutr. First published August 4, 2010. doi: 10.3945/ajcn.2009.29146. Consulted April 12, 2015.

- Saslow, L. R. et al. An online intervention comparing a very low-carbohydrate ketogenic diet and lifestyle recommendations versus a plate method diet in overweight individuals with type 2 diabetes: A randomized controlled trial. J Med Internet Res. February 13, 2017;19(2):e36.

- Roberts, M. N. et al. A ketogenic diet extends longevity and healthspan in adult mice. Cell Metab. September 5, 2017;26(3):539-546:e5.

- Liu, Y. M., Wang, H. S. Medium-chain triglyceride ketogenic diet, an effective treatment for drug-resistant epilepsy and a comparison with other ketogenic diets. Biomed J. January-February 2013;36(1):9-15.

Fructose

- Lustig, R. H. Fructose: Metabolic, hedonic, and societal parallels with ethanol. J Am Diet Assoc. 2010; 110(9):1307-1321.

- Beck-Nielsen, H. et al. Impaired cellular insulin binding and insulin sensitivity induced by high-fructose feeding in normal subjects. Am J Clin Nutr. February 1980;33(2):273-278.

- Stanhope, K. L,. et al. Consuming fructose-sweetened, not glucose-sweetened, beverages increases visceral adiposity and lipids and decreases insulin sensitivity in overweight/obese humans. JCI. 2009;119(5):1322-1334.

- Bizeau, M. E. and M. J. Pagliassotti. Hepatic adaptations to sucrose and fructose. Metabolism. 2005;54(9):1189-1201.

- Faeh, D. et al. Effect of fructose overfeeding and fish oil administration on hepatic de novo lipogenesis and insulin sensitivity in healthy men. Diabetes. 2005;54(7):1907-1913.

- Basu, S. et al. The relationship of sugar to population-level diabetes prevalence: An econometric analysis of repeated cross-sectional data. PLoS One. 2013;8(2):e57873.

- Ridgeway, L. USC News. High fructose corn syrup linked to diabetes. November 28, 2012. Available at: https://news. usc. edu/44415/high-fructose-corn-syrup-linked-to-diabetes/. Consulted June 6, 2017.

- Goran, M. I. et al. High fructose corn syrup and diabetes prevalence: A global perspective. Glob Pub Health. 2013;8(1):55-64.

- Grundy, S. M. et al. Diagnosis and management of the metabolic syndrome: An American Heart Association/National Heart, Lung, and Blood Institute Scientific Statement. Circulation. October 25, 2005;112(17):2735-2752.

- Ginsberg, H. N. and P. R. MacCallum. The obesity, metabolic syndrome, and type 2 diabetes mellitus pandemic: Part I. Increased cardiovascular disease risk and the importance of atherogenic dyslipidemia in persons with the metabolic syndrome and type 2 diabetes mellitus. Cardiometab Syndr. Spring 2009;4(2):113-119.

- Ibarra-Reynoso, L. D. R., López-Lemus, H. L., Garay-Sevilla, M. E. and J. M. Malacara. Effect of restriction of foods with high fructose corn syrup content on metabolic indices and fatty liver in obese children. Obes Facts. August 5, 2017;10(4):332-40.

- Ruanpeng, D., Thongprayoon, C., Cheungpasitporn, W. and T. Harindhanavudhi. Sugar and artificially-sweetened beverages linked to obesity: A systematic review and meta-analysis. QJM. April 11, 2017.

- Greenwood, D. C., Threapleton, D. E., Evans, C. E. et al. Association between sugar-sweetened and artificially sweetened soft drinks and type 2 diabetes: Systematic review and dose-response meta-analysis of prospective studies. Br J Nutr. September 14, 2014;112(5):725-734.

- Wijarnpreecha, K., Thongprayoon, C., Edmonds, P. J. and W. Cheungpasitporn. Associations of sugar-and artificially sweetened soda with nonalcoholic fatty liver disease: A systematic review and meta-analysis. QJM. July 2016;109(7):461-466.

- Cheungpasitporn, W., Thongprayoon, C., O'Corragain, O. A., Edmonds, P. J., Kittanamongkolchai, W. and S. B. Erickson. Associations of sugar-sweetened and artificially sweetened soda with chronic kidney disease: A systematic review and meta-analysis. Nephrology (Carlton). December 2014;19(12):791-797.

- Vos, M. B. and J. E. Lavine. Dietary fructose in nonalcoholic fatty liver disease. Hepatology. June 2013;57(6):2525-2531.

- Bray, G. A., Nielsen, S. J. and B. M. Popkin. Consumption of high-fructose corn syrup in beverages may play a role in the epidemic of obesity. Am J Clin Nutr. April 2004;79(4):537-543.

Artificial sweeteners

- Maher, T. J. and R. J. Wurtman. Possible neurologic effects of aspartame, a widely used food additive. Environ Health Perspect. November 1987;75:53-57.

- Wang, Q. P. , Lin, Y. Q., Zhang, L. et al. Sucralose promotes food intake through NPY and a neuronal fasting response. Cell Metab. July 12, 2016;24(1):75-90.

- Phillips, K. M., Carlsen, M. H. and R. Blomhoff. Total antioxidant content of alternatives to refined sugar. J Am Diet Assoc. January 2009;109(1):64-71.

- Clay, J. World Agriculture and the Environment: A Commodity-By-Commodity Guide to Impacts and Practices. Washington, DC: Island Press; March 1, 2004.

- Elizabeth, K. UNCW professors study Splenda in Cape Fear River. Star News Online. March 10, 2013.

- Wu-Smart, J. and M. Spivak. Sub-lethal effects of dietary neonicotinoid insecticide exposure on honey bee queen fecundity and colony development. Sci Rep. August 26, 2016;6:32108.

- Tey, S. L., Salleh, N. B., Henry, J. and C. G. Forde. Effects of aspartame-, monk fruit-, stevia- and sucrose-sweetened beverages on postprandial glucose, insulin and energy intake. Int J Obes (London). March 2017;41(3):450-457.

- Swithers, S. E. and T. L. Davidson. A role for sweet taste: Calorie predictive relations in energy regulation by rats. Behav Neurosci. February 2008;122(1):161-173.

- Feijó, F. de M., Ballard, C. R. , Foletto, K. C. et al. Saccharin and aspartame, compared with sucrose, induce greater weight gain in adult Wistar rats, at similar total caloric intake levels. Appetite. January 2013;60(1):203-207.

- Borges, M. C., Louzada, M. L., De Sa, T. H. et al. Artificially sweetened beverages and the response to the global obesity crisis. PLoS Med. January 3, 2017;14(1):e1002195.

- Hootman, K. C., Trezzi, J. P., Kraemer, L. et al. Erythritol is a pentose-phosphate pathway metabolite and associated with adiposity gain in young adults. Proc Natl Acad Sci U S A. May 23, 2017;114(21):E4233-E4240. doi: 10.1073/pnas.1620079114.

- Nettleton, J. A., Lutsey, P. L., Wang, Y. et al. Diet soda intake and risk of incident metabolic syndrome and type 2 diabetes in the Multi-Ethnic Study of Atherosclerosis (mesa). Diabetes Care. 2009;32(4):688-94.

- Soffritti, M., Belpoggi, F., Manservigi, M. et al. Aspartame administered in feed, beginning prenatally through life span, induces cancers of the liver and lung in male Swiss mice. Am J Ind Med. December 2010;53(12):1197-1206.

- Suez, J., Korem, T., Zeevi, D. et al. Artificial sweeteners induce glucose intolerance by altering the gut microbiota. Nature. 2014;514(7521):181-186.

- Van Opstal, A. M. Dietary sugars and non-caloric sweeteners elicit different homeostatic and hedonic responses in the brain. Nutrition. September 13, 2018;60:80-86. doi: 10.1016/j.nut.2018.09.004.

- Romo-Romo, A. Sucralose decreases insulin sensitivity in healthy subjects: A randomized controlled trial. Am J Clin Nutr. September 1, 2018;108(3):485-491.
- Kramer, H. The Millennial Physician and the Obesity Epidemic: A Tale of Sugar-Sweetened Beverages. Clin J Am Soc Nephrol. January 7, 2019;14(1):4-6. doi: 10.2215/ CJN.13851118. Electronic publication: December 27, 2018.

Dairy

- Danby, F. W. Acne, dairy and cancer. Dermatoendocrinol. January-February 2009;1(1):12-16.
- Duarte-Salles, T. Dairy products and risk of hepatocellular carcinoma: The European Prospective Investigation into Cancer and Nutrition. Int J Cancer. October 1, 2014;135(7):1662-1672.
- Larsson, S. C. Milk, milk products and lactose intake and ovarian cancer risk: A meta-analysis of epidemiological studies. Int J Cancer. January 15, 2006;118(2):431-441.
- Harrison, S. et al. Does milk intake promote prostate cancer initiation or progression via effects on insulin-like growth factors (IGFs)? A systematic review and meta-analysis. Cancer Causes Control. June 2017;28(6):497-528.
- Günther, A. L. Early Diet and Later Cancer Risk: Prospective Associations of Dietary Patterns During Critical Periods of Childhood with the GH-IGF Axis, Insulin Resistance and Body Fatness in Younger Adulthood. Nutr Cancer. 2015;67(6):877-892.
- Chan, J. M. Dairy products, calcium, and vitamin D and risk of prostate cancer. Epidemiol Rev. 2001;23(1):87-92.
- Ludwig, D. S. and W. C. Willett. Three daily servings of reduced-fat milk: An evidence-based recommendation? JAMA Pediatr. September 2013;167(9):788–789.

- Danby, F. W. Acne, dairy and cancer: The 5alpha-P link. Dermatoendocrinol. January 2009;1(1):12-16.
- Bischoff-Ferrari, H. A., Dawson-Hughes, B., Baron, J. A. et al. Milk intake and risk of hip fracture in men and women: A meta-analysis of prospective cohort studies. J Bone Miner Res. 2011;26(4):833-839.
- Heyman, M. B. Lactose intolerance in infants, children and adolescents. Pediatrics. September 2006;118(3):1279-1286.
- Berkey, C. S., Rockett, H. R., Willett, W. C. et al. Milk, dairy fat, dietary calcium and weight gain: A longitudinal study of adolescents. Arch Pediatr Adolesc Med. June 2005;159(6):543-550.
- Mozaffarian, D., Hao, T., Rimm, E. B. et al. Changes in diet and lifestyle and long-term weight gain in women and men. N Engl J Med. 2011;364(25):2392-2404.
- The Dairy Practices Council. Guideline for Vitamin A & D Fortification of Fluid Milk. http://phpa.dhmh.maryland.gov/OEHFP/OFPCHS/Milk/Shared%20Documents/DPC053_Vitamin_ AD_Fortification_Fluid_Milk.pdf. July 2001.
- Dietitians for Professional Integrity. How industry lobbying shapes the dietary guidelines. http://integritydietitians.org/2015/11/18/how-industry-lobbying-shapes-the-dietary-guidelines/. November 18, 2015.
- Lanou, A. J. Should dairy be recommended as part of a healthy vegetarian diet? Counterpoint. Am J Clin Nutr. May 2009;89(5):1638S-1642S.
- Feskanich, D., Willett, W. C., Stampfer, M. J. et al. Milk, dietary calcium, and bone fractures in women: A 12-year prospective study. Am J Public Health. 1997;87:992-997.
- Winzenberg, T., Shaw, K., Fryer, J. et al. Effects of calcium supplementation on bone density in healthy children: Meta-analysis of randomized controlled trials. BMJ. October 14, 2006;333(7572):775.

- Feskanich, D., Willett, W. C. and G. A. Colditz. Calcium, vitamin D, milk consumption, and hip fractures: A prospective study among postmenopausal women. Am J Clin Nutr. February 2003;77(2):504-511.

- Friedrich, N., Thuesen, B., Jorgensen, T. et al. The association between IGF-1 and insulin resistance: A general population study in Danish adults. Diabetes Care. April 2012;35(4):768-773.

- Yakoob, M. Y., Shi, P., Willett, W. C. et al. Circulating biomarkers of dairy fat and risk of incident diabetes mellitus among men and women in the United States in two large prospective cohorts. Circulation. April 26, 2016;133(17):1645- 1654.

- Carroccio, A., Brusca, I., Mansueto, P. et al. Fecal assays detect hypersensitivity to cow's milk protein and gluten in adults with irritable bowel syndrome. Clin Gastroenterol Hepatol. November 2011;9(11):965-971.

- Howchwallner, H., Schulmeister, U., Swoboda, I. et al. Cow's milk allergy: From allergens to new forms of diagnosis, therapy and prevention. Methods. March 2014;66(1):22-33.

- Katta, R. and M. Schlichte. Diet and dermatitis: Food triggers. J Clin Aesthet Dermatol. March 2014;7(3):30-36.

- Lill, C., Loader, B., Seemann, R. et al. Milk allergy is frequent in patients with chronic sinusitis and nasal polyposis. Am J Rhinol Allergy. November-December 2011;25(6):e221-e224.

Gluten

- Serena, G., Camhi, S., Sturgeon, C., Yan, Sh. and Fasano, A. The Role of Gluten in Celiac Disease and Type 1 Diabetes, Nutrients. September 2015;7(9): 7143-7162.

- Catassi, C. Diagnosis of Non-Celiac Gluten Sensitivity (NCGS): The Salerno Experts' Criteria. Nutrients. June 2015;7(6):4966-4977.

- Sapone, A. Spectrum of gluten-related disorders: Consensus on new nomenclature and classification. BMC Med. 2012;10:13. Electronic publication: February 7, 2012.
- Catassi, C. Non-Celiac Gluten Sensitivity: The New Frontier of Gluten Related Disorders. Nutrients. October 2013;5(10):3839-3853. Electronic publication: September 26, 2013.
- Samsel, A. and S. Seneff. Glyphosate, pathways to modern diseases II: Celiac sprue and gluten intolerance. Interdisciplinary Toxicology. 2013;6(4):159-184.
- Samsel, A. and S. Seneff. Glyphosate's suppression of cytochrome P450 enzymes and amino acid biosynthesis by the gut microbiome: Pathways to modern diseases. Entropy. 2013;15:1416- 1463.
- Hyman, M. Food: What the Heck Should I Eat? Little, Brown and Company. Kindle edition.
- Jackson, J. R. Neurologic and Psychiatric Manifestations of Celiac Disease and Gluten Sensitivity. Psychiatr Q. Author's manuscript; available at PMC, May 2, 2013.
- Rostami, K. Gluten-Free Diet Indications, Safety, Quality, Labels, and Challenges. Nutrients. August 2017;9(8):846.
- Uhde, M., Ajamian, M., Caio, G. et al. Intestinal cell damage and systemic immune activation in individuals reporting sensitivity to wheat in the absence of coeliac disease. Gut. 2016;65:1930-1937.

- Rubio-Tapia, A., Kyle, R. A., Kaplan, E. L. et al. Increased prevalence and mortality in undiagnosed celiac disease. Gastroenterology. July 2009;137(1):88-93.
- Sturgeon, C. and A. Fasano. Zonulin, a regulator of epithelial and endothelial barrier functions, and its involvement in chronic inflammatory diseases. Tissue Barriers. October 21, 2016;4(4):e1251384.

Chapter 7
Physical activity

Working out on an empty stomach

- Achten, J., Gleeson, M. and A. E. Jeukendrup. Determination of the exercise intensity that elicits maximal fat oxidation. Med Sci Sports Exerc. 2002;34(1):92-97.
- Goedecke, J. H., St Clair Gibson, A., Grobler, L., Collins, M., Noakes, T. D. and E. V. Lambert. Determinants of the variability in respiratory exchange ratio at rest and during exercise in trained athletes. Am J Physiol Endocrinol Metab. 2000;279(6):E1325-E1334.
- Venables, M. C., Achten, J. and A. E. Jeukendrup. Determinants of fat oxidation during exercise in healthy men and women: a cross-sectional study. J Appl Physiol. 2005;98(1):160-167.
- McKenzie, E., Holbrook, T., Williamson, K., Royer, C., Valberg, S., Hinchcliff, K., José-Cunilleras, E., Nelson, S., Willard, M., Davis, M. Recovery of muscle glycogen concentrations in sled dogs during prolonged exercise. Med Sci Sports Exerc. 2005;37(8):1307- 1312.

- Phinney, S. The Art and Science of Low Carbohydrate Performance. Beyond Obesity LLC. Kindle edition.
- McKenzie, E. C., Hinchcliff, K. W., Valberg, S. J., Williamson, K. K., Payton, M. E. and M. S. Davis. Assessment of alterations in triglyceride and glycogen concentrations in muscle tissue of Alaskan sled dogs during repetitive prolonged exercise. Am J Vet Res. 2008;69(8):1097-1103.
- Volek, J. S., Quann, E. E. and C. E. Forsythe. Low carbohydrate diets promote a more favorable body composition than low fat diets. Strength and Conditioning Journal. 2010;32(1):42-47.
- Cahill Jr., G. F. and T. T. Aoki. Alternate fuel utilization by brain. In: Passonneau, J. V. et al (eds.). Cerebral Metabolism and Neural Function. Williams & Wilkins, Baltimore, 1980. Pp 234-242.
- Forsythe, C. E., Phinney, S. D., Fernández, M. L., Quann, E. E., Wood, R. J., Bibus, D. M., Kraemer, W. J, Feinman, R. D. and J. S. Volek. Comparison of low fat and low carbohydrate diets on circulating fatty acid composition and markers of inflammation. Lipids. 2008;43(1):65-77.
- Jarrett, S. G., Milder, J. B., Liang, L. P. and M. Patel. The ketogenic diet increases mitochondrial glutathione levels. J Neurochem. 2008;106(3):1044-1051.
- Sahlin, K., Shabalina, I. G., Mattsson, C. M., Bakkman, L., Fernstrom, M., Rozhdestvenskaya, Z., Enqvist, J. K., Nedergaard, J., Ekblom, B. and M. Tonkonogi. Ultraendurance exercise increases the production of reactive oxygen species in isolated mitochondria from human skeletal muscle. J Appl Physiol. 2010;108 (4):780-787.

Part three
The metabolic miracle

- Foster-Powell, K., Holt, S. H. A. and J. C. Brand-Miller. International Table of Glycemic Index and Glycemic Load Values: 2002. American Journal of Clinical Nutrition. January 2002;76:5-56. http://ajcn.nutrition.org/content/76/1/5.full.pdf.

- Frei, B., Ames, B. N., Blumberg, J. B. and W. C. Willett. Enough Is Enough. Annals of Internal Medicine. June 3, 2014;160(11):807.

- Solon-Biet, S. M. The Ratio of Macronutrients, Not Caloric Intake, Dictates Cardiometabolic Health, Aging, and Longevity in Ad Libitum-Fed Mice. Cell Metabolism. March 4, 2014;19(3):418-430.

- Levine, M. and V. D. Longo. Low Protein Intake Is Associated with a Major Reduction in IGF-1, Cancer, and Overall Mortality in the 65 and Younger but Not Older Population. Cell Metabolism. March 4, 2014;19(3):407-417.

- Song, M., Fung, T. T., Hu, F. B., Willett, W. C., Longo, V. D., Chan, A. T. and Giovannucci E. L. Association of Animal and Plant Protein Intake With All-Cause and Cause-Specific Mortality. JAMA Internal Medicine. 2016;176(10):1453-1463.

- Pollack, M. Insulin and Insulin-Like Growth Factor Signaling in Neoplasia. Nature Reviews Cancer. December 2008;8(12):915-928.

- Yang, M. U. y T. B. Van Itallie. Composition of Weight Lost During Short-Term Weight Reduction: Metabolic Responses of Obese Subjects to Starvation and Low-Calorie Ketogenic and Nonketogenic Diets. Journal of Clinical Investigation. September 1976;58(3):722-730.

- Willett, W. C., Dietz, W. H. and G. A. Colditz. Guidelines for Healthy Weight. New England Journal of Medicine. August 1999;341:427-434.

- Pischon, T., Boeing, H., Hoffmann, K. et al. General and Abdominal Adiposity and Risk of Death in Europe. New England Journal of Medicine. November 13, 2008;359:2105-2120.

- Barnosky, A. R., Hoody, K. K., Unterman, T. G. and K. A. Varady, Intermittent Fasting vs. Daily Calorie Restriction for Type 2 Diabetes Prevention: A Review of Human Findings. Translation Research. October 2014,164(4): 302-311.

- Bangalore, S., Fayyad, R., Laskey, R., DeMicco, D. A., Messerli, F. H. and D. D. Waters. Body Weight Outcomes in Coronary Disease. New England Journal of Medicine. April 6, 2017;(376):1332- 1340. doi: 10.1056/NEJMoa1606148.

- Hall, K. D. Diet Versus Exercise in "The Biggest Loser" Weight Loss Competition. Obesity. 21:957–959. doi: 10.1002/oby.20065.

- Colman, R. J., Anderson, R. M. et al. Caloric Restriction Delays Disease Onset and Mortality in Rhesus Monkeys. Science. July 10, 2009;325(5937).

- Colman, R. J., Beasley, T. M. et al. Caloric Restriction Reduces Age-Related and All-Cause Mortality in Rhesus Monkeys. Nature. April 2014;325(5937):201-204.

- Sofi, F., Macchi C. et al. Mediterranean Diet and Health Status: An Updated Meta-Analysis and a Proposal for a Literature-Based Adherence Score. Public Health Nutrition December 2014;17(12):2769-2782.

- Bendinelli B., Masala G. et al. Fruit, Vegetables, and Olive Oil and Risk of Coronary Heart Disease in Italian Women: The EPICOR Study. American Journal of Clinical Nutrition. February 2011;93(2):275-283.

- Buckland, G., Travier, N. et al. Olive Oil Intake and Breast Cancer Risk in the Mediterranean Countries of the European Prospective Investigation into Cancer and Nutrition Study. International Journal of Cancer. 2012;131:2465-2469.

- Bao, Y., Han, J. et al. Association of Nut Consumption with Total and Cause-Specific Mortality. New England Journal of Medicine. November 2013;369:2001-2011.

- Bendinelli, B., G. Masala, et al. Fruit, Vegetables, and Olive Oil and Risk of Coronary Heart Disease in Italian Women: The EPICOR Study. American Journal of Clinical Nutrition. February 2011;93(2):275-283.

- Buckland, G., Travier, N. et al. Olive Oil Intake and Breast Cancer Risk in the Mediterranean Countries of the European Prospective Investigation into Cancer and Nutrition Study. International Journal of Cancer. 2012;131:2465-2469.

- Kerndt, P. R. et al. Fasting: the history, pathophysiology and complications. West J Med. November 1982;137(5):379-399.

- Harvie, M. N. et al. The effects of intermittent or continuous energy restriction on weight loss and metabolic disease risk markers. Int J Obes (London). May 2011;35(5):714-727.

- Klempel, M. C. et al. Intermittent fasting combined with calorie restriction is effective for weight loss and cardio-protection in obese women. Nutr J. 2012;11:98. doi: 10.1186/1475-2891-11-98. Consulted April 8, 2015.

- Thomson, T. J. et al. Treatment of obesity by total fasting for up to 249 days. Lancet. November 5, 1966;2(7471):992-996.